Earn CME while you learn!

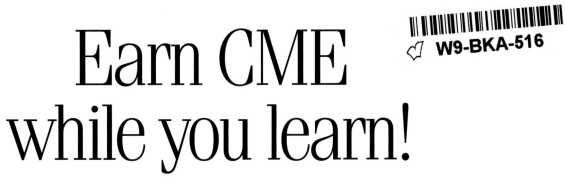

W9-BKA-516

Up to 90 hours of CME credit available with the MedStudy Internal Medicine Review Core Curriculum - 10th Edition

The 2003/2004 10th Edition MedStudy Internal Medicine Review Core Curriculum offers you the opportunity to earn up to 90 hours of Category 1 credit towards the AMA Physician's Recognition Award.

This CME credit is provided through the Tulane University Health Sciences Center in a CME joint sponsorship arrangement with MedStudy. To apply for your CME credit, you must complete the **Verification of Credit** form found immediately following the next page. Then submit that completed form along with the $40 CME fee to the Center for Continuing Education at Tulane University Health Sciences Center. All the necessary contact information is included on the **Verification of Credit** form. Please note that CME credit is available only to the original purchaser of this product, and issuance of CME credit is subject to verification of product ownership.

The Release Date for the MedStudy Internal Medicine Review Core Curriculum is December 1, 2002. To be eligible for CME credit, you must study the content of the Core Curriculum and submit your **Verification of Credit** form no later than December 1, 2004 (Expiration Date).

Disclosure Statement

Tulane University Health Sciences Center adheres to the ACCME's Essential Areas and Their Elements and Criteria regarding industry support of continuing medical education. Disclosures of faculty and commercial relationships have been documented below. Faculty have openly disclosed inclusion of discussion of any off-label, experimental, or investigational use of drugs or devices in their presentations and/or have indicated an affiliation with organizations which have interests related to content of this activity.

Norton Greenberger, MD, has disclosed that he is a consultant for McNeil Consumer Pharmaceuticals and serves as a speaker for Centocor and Astra Merck
Robert A. Balk, MD, has disclosed that he serves as a speaker for GlaxoSmithKline, Ortho-Biotech, and Eli Lilly
Paul Sutej, MD, has disclosed that he serves as a speaker for Merck, Pfizer, Aventis, and Pharmacia
Robert Richards, MD, has disclosed that he receives grant/research support from GlaxoSmithKline and serves as a speaker for Wyeth-Ayerst, Pfizer, and Novo Nordisk
Alan Morganstein, MD, has disclosed that he is a consultant for GlaxoSmithKline, Ortho-McNeil, Pfizer, Abbott, and Ortho-Biotech and serves as a speaker for GlaxoSmithKline, Ortho-McNeil, Pfizer, and Abbott

Accreditation

This activity has been planned and implemented in accordance with the Essential Areas and Policies of the Accreditation Council for Continuing Medical Education through the joint sponsorship of Tulane University Health Sciences Center and MedStudy. Tulane University Health Sciences Center is accredited by the Accreditation Council for Continuing Medical Education (ACCME) to provide continuing medical education for physicians.

Tulane University Health Sciences Center designates this educational activity for a maximum of 90 hours in Category 1 credit towards the AMA Physician's Recognition Award. Each physician should claim only those hours of credit that he/she actually spent in the educational activity.

Tulane University Health Sciences Center presents this activity for educational purposes only and does not endorse any product or content of presentation. Participants are expected to utilize their own expertise and judgment while engaged in the practice of medicine. The content of the presentation is provided solely by presenters who have been selected because of their recognized expertise.

DISCLOSURE STATEMENT

2003/2004 10th Edition MedStudy
Internal Medicine Review Core Curriculum

Tulane University Health Sciences Center adheres to the ACCME's Essential Areas and Their Elements and Criteria regarding industry support of continuing medical education. Disclosures of authors/contributors/reviewers and commercial relationships have been documented below.

I.   Contributors/Reviewers have openly disclosed inclusion of discussion of any off-label, experimental, or investigational use of drugs or devices in their submitted and/or reviewed content and have indicated an affiliation with organizations which have interests related to the content of this product:

Contributor	Affiliation/Disclosure(s)
Norton Greenberger, MD	Consultant - McNeil Consumer Pharmaceuticals
	Speaker - Centocor, Astra Merck
Robert A. Balk, MD	Speaker - GlaxoSmithKline, Ortho-Biotech, Eli Lilly
Paul Sutej, MD	Speaker - Merck, Pfizer, Aventis, Pharmacia
Robert Richards, MD	Grant/Research Support - GlaxoSmithKline
	Speaker - Wyeth-Ayerst, Pfizer, Novo Nordisk
Alan Morganstein, MD	Consultant - GlaxoSmithKline, Ortho-McNeil, Pfizer, Abbott, Ortho-Biotech
	Speaker - GlaxoSmithKline, Ortho-McNeil, Pfizer, Abbott

II.   The following contributor(s) have documented they have nothing to disclose:

Robert A. Hannaman. MD
Frederic Kraemer, MD
J. Thomas Cross, MD
N. Kevin Krane, MD

III.   The following contributor(s) have received forms but have not provided disclosure information at production time:

Margery Scott, MD
David Abrams, MD
Harold S. Novey, MD, FACP
Steven Karceski, MD

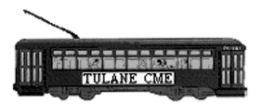

MedStudy Internal Medicine Review Core Curriculum
CME Application

Center for Continuing Education
Tulane University Health Sciences Center
1430 Tulane Avenue, TB-51
New Orleans, Louisiana 70112-2699
(504) 588-5466; (504) 584-1779 FAX

IMPORTANT NOTE: You must complete both sides of this form and submit to TUHSC-CCE to receive CME credit. CME credit is available only to the original purchaser of this product. Issuance of a CME Certificate is subject to verification of product ownership.

Verification of Credit/Attendance
MedStudy 10th Edition Internal Medicine Review Core Curriculum

Release date: December1, 2002

This activity has been planned and implemented in accordance with the Essential Areas and Policies of the Accreditation Council for Continuing Medical Education through the joint sponsorship of Tulane University Health Sciences Center and MedStudy. Tulane University Health Sciences Center is accredited by the Accreditation Council for Continuing Medical Education (ACCME) to provide continuing medical education for physicians.

Tulane University Health Sciences Center designates this educational activity for a maximum of 90 hours in Category 1 credit towards the AMA Physician's Recognition Award. Each physician should claim only those hours of credit that he/she actually spent in the educational activity.

My signature on this document certifies my review and participation in the MedStudy CME Internal Medicine Review Core Curriculum. I have logged _____hours and claim the same for AMA/PRA Category 1 CME credit (maximum of 90 hours).

Signature _____ Date _____

Printed Name: _____

Street Address: _____

City/State/Zip Code: _____

Telephone:_____ Fax:_____

Email: _____ Specialty _____

CME processing fee: $40
Payment method: ___ Check or money order (payable to TUHSC-CCE)
                       ___ Visa   ___ MasterCard
               FAX (credit card payments) (504) 584-1779
               Mail: Tulane University Health Sciences Center
                        Center for Continuing Education, TB-51
                        1430 Tulane Avenue
                        New Orleans, LA 70112-2699

Card # _____ Expiration Date _____

Authorized signature _____

Learning Activity Evaluation

MedStudy Internal Medicine Review Core Curriculum

Using the following scale, please respond to the statements below by circling the appropriate letter:
A=Strongly Agree   B=Agree   C=Not Applicable   D=Disagree   E=Strongly Disagree

OBJECTIVES

1. To what extent were the following objectives met?

After studying this program, you should be more confident in:

Grasping subjects relevant to the depth and scope of the ABIM certifying or recertifying exam	A	B	C	D	E
Discussing accepted approaches to the diagnosis and therapy of conditions commonly seen by Internal Medicine practitioners, and also remedying any weaknesses in Internal Medicine	A	B	C	D	E
Generating a comprehensive differential diagnosis based on a set of presenting signs and symptoms	A	B	C	D	E
Effectively narrowing the differential diagnosis list by utilizing appropriate laboratory studies, scans, etc.	A	B	C	D	E

OVERALL

2. This activity is balanced and free of commercial bias	A	B	C	D	E
3. My professional knowledge and skills were updated	A	B	C	D	E
4. I feel better prepared to sit for a competency examination	A	B	C	D	E
5. I was able to develop a strategy for self-study prior to the exam	A	B	C	D	E

6. Do you feel the content, organization and format in these books is a viable mode of instructional delivery?
  __ Yes   __ No   __ Prefer other

7. The activity content was:
  __ Satisfactory   __ Too advanced   __ Too basic

8. What did you find to be the most valuable component of this activity?

_____

_____

_____

_____

Please FAX or MAIL this completed form using fax number/address from side 1.

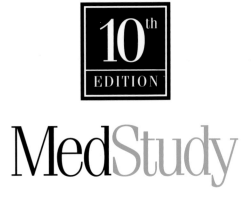

MedStudy

The Internal Medicine Review

Book 1 of 5

Topics in this volume:

Gastroenterology

Infectious Disease

Authored by Robert A. Hannaman, MD

This material is authored by Robert A. Hannaman, MD
Publisher: MedStudy

MEDSTUDY
1761 South 8th Street, Building H1
Colorado Springs, Colorado 80906
(800) 841-0547

Table of Contents

Gastroenterology

Infectious Disease **TOC** on next page

Table of Contents

Infectious Disease

MedStudy

The Internal Medicine Review

Gastroenterology

Authored by Robert A. Hannaman, MD

Many thanks to

Norton J. Greenberger, MD
Clinical Professor of Medicine
Brigham and Women's Hospital
Boston, Massachusetts

Gastroenterology Advisor

ENDOSCOPY

Contraindications to GI endoscopy include a recent MI, combative patient, and intestinal perforation.

Esophagogastroduodenoscopy (EGD) is the procedure of choice for:

1) evaluation of painful swallowing (odynophagia)
2) determining presence of a peptic ulcer—either instead of an UGI or when the UGI is equivocal or negative—and always before PUD surgery
   3) workup of GERD if initial treatment fails or if there are alarm signals (see GERD)
   4) UGI bleed workup
   5) workup of GI disease during pregnancy
   6) for dysphagia (*after* the barium swallow!)
   7) prn for evaluation of an ingested foreign body
   8) for persistent dyspepsia (a normal EGD is necessary for diagnosis of non-ulcer dyspepsia)

Endoscopic retrograde cholangiopancreatography (ERCP): Sixty percent of patients have an elevated amylase after ERCP and acute pancreatitis occurs in 2-8%. Patients with possible bile duct obstruction should be treated with antibiotics before ERCP. Indications for ERCP are unclear, but it is often used in three situations: it is the best method for finding otherwise undetectable common duct stones and for determining the cause of pancreatic duct obstruction; it also may be needed to diagnose chronic pancreatitis. ERCP is contraindicated in acute pancreatitis except in the following conditions: a) impacted gallstones, b) lack of clinical improvement of a non-alcoholic acute pancreatitis, and c) cholangitis.

Retrograde cholangiography visualizes the bile tract (percutaneous transhepatic cholangiography [PTC], U/S, CT scan, and PIPIDA scans are also used). Retrograde pancreatography is used to visualize the pancreatic duct. Colonoscopy is discussed later.

ESOPHAGUS

DYSPHAGIA

Note: problems of the esophagus often present with dysphagia. There are two types of dysphagia:

1) Transfer dysphagia resulting from difficulty transferring food from the mouth to the esophagus. Caused by oral-pharyngeal muscle dysfunction as in CVA, ALS, etc. (see neurologic dysfunction below) and sometimes with a Zenker diverticulum.
2) Transport dysphagia: which is trouble with transporting the food from the upper esophagus to the stomach. It has endogenous or exogenous causes.

The barium swallow is the first test usually performed in the workup of dysphagia. It is done before endoscopy because
1) there is a risk of perforation when endoscoping a patient with a diverticula,

2) information from the barium swallow may preclude the need for endoscopy. Endoscopy is then done if indicated.

Motility studies are usually done if these two tests are negative. (Again, workup of dysphagia: 1 = barium swallow, 2 = endoscopy, 3 = motility studies.)

ACHALASIA

Achalasia consists of the absence or failure of esophageal smooth muscle peristalsis and increased tonus of the lower esophageal sphincter (LES). Patients often regurgitate food several hours after eating. During a presurgical exam, keep in mind that these patients are at high risk for aspiration. Chagas disease is seen in South America—it causes achalasia, cardiomyopathy, and megacolon.

Diagnosis: First, as with virtually all dysphagias, do a barium swallow—in this case it shows a dilated, fluid-filled esophagus with a smooth, tapered ("bird's beak") narrowing at the GE junction. Manometry further clarifies the diagnosis with the findings noted above (failure of peristalsis and increased LES tone). Endoscopy is necessary to confirm the diagnosis because it is necessary to rule out a secondary achalasia (see next) due to cancer or lymphoma. (3 tests: 1-Barium swallow, 2-manometry, 3-endoscopy).

Suspect secondary achalasia (cancer, lymphoma) when: Onset after age 60, < 6 month duration of symptoms, and weight loss.

Treatment for achalasia is focused at opening the LES. Usual treatment is pneumatic dilation of the LES in which a large 4cm balloon is inflated within the LES and tears the sphincter open. There is a 5% risk of perforation. Surgical myotomy is also very effective and can now be done via laparoscope. Botulinum toxin is effective in 65% but repeat therapy is required in 1-2 years—it is an alternative therapy in high-risk patients. Calcium channel blockers and nitrates have been used in the past with, at best, temporary partial relief.

ESOPHAGEAL SPASM

Diffuse esophageal spasm (DES) is a simultaneous non-peristaltic contraction of the esophagus, often precipitated by cold or carbonated liquids. It is an uncommon disorder and is therefore a rare cause of noncardiac chest pain. Barium swallow is usually normal but may show the classic corkscrew pattern. Manometry confirms the diagnosis by revealing intermittent simultaneous (nonperistaltic) contractions. LES pressure may be low, normal, or high (i.e., nonspecific). There are no good studies on treatment of DES—generally calcium channel blockers, muscle relaxers, and nitrates are used. Symptoms are often self-limited.

NUTCRACKER ESOPHAGUS

Nutcracker esophagus was thought to be another cause of chest pain. Manometry shows intermittent high pressure indicating strong peristaltic contractions. Note: these contractions are

notes

not always associated with chest pain, nor is the chest pain always associated with the contractions! This entity is now thought to be more of an incidental finding of limited clinical significance. Similar findings and symptoms can be caused by gastroesophageal reflux so this should be ruled out with a 24 hr esophageal pH study.

ANATOMIC OBSTRUCTION

Anatomic obstruction causes a progressive dysphagia—initially to solids and then to liquids when severe. In younger patients, it is usually caused by a Schatzki ring (lower esophageal ring), whereas in older patients it is usually due to cancer [pg 123 #366, 368, 369]! Patients with a lower esophageal ring always have hiatal hernia but it is unknown if reflux plays a role. Other causes of anatomic obstruction include:
• peptic strictures due to chronic GE reflux
• mediastinal masses
• Plummer-Vinson syndrome
• lye strictures
• Zenker's diverticulum

Plummer-Vinson syndrome is iron deficiency in association with a symptomatic hypopharyngeal web (causing symptoms of glossitis); it is found most often in middle-aged women. Risk of squamous cell cancer is increased in these patients.

Although all causes of anatomic obstruction are progressive, rings typically cause intermittent symptoms while symptoms due to cancer and stricture are relentlessly progressive. 75% of the circumference must be involved before symptoms occur.

Treat lower esophageal ring with pneumatic dilation.

NEUROLOGIC DYSFUNCTION

Neurologic problems involving the swallowing and/or esophageal peristaltic mechanism cause dysphagia to solids and liquids. Examples from above are achalasia and diffuse esophageal spasm. Other examples include CVA, Parkinsonism, bulbar palsy (lower motor neuron—ALS, MS) and pseudobulbar palsy (upper motor neuron—ALS). Either of these may be seen as variants of early amyotrophic lateral sclerosis (ALS) whereas multiple sclerosis may cause only bulbar palsy. Bulbar palsy causes dysphagia due to weakness, whereas pseudobulbar palsy causes dysphagia due to disordered contractions. Any type of dysphagia can cause aspiration. This aspiration is often well tolerated and does not need treatment unless there are pulmonary problems. If aspiration is suspected, a three-phase barium swallow should be done to confirm the diagnosis. Tracheostomy does not often cure chronic aspiration.

SCLERODERMA

Progressive systemic sclerosis (PSS; scleroderma) is the most common connective tissue disease involving the esophagus. Over 80% of PSS patients have involvement of the esopha-

gus! It causes reduced to absent peristaltic contractions (like achalasia) in addition to a low LES pressure (unlike achalasia). The clinical picture is a neuromuscular one of progressive dysphagia to solids and liquids. The low LES pressure causes severe GERD (see below). Poly/ dermatomyositis may cause similar effects.

ESOPHAGITIS

Esophagitis often presents with odynophagia (painful swallowing). In the immunosuppressed, especially consider infection: *Candida*, Herpes Simplex, CMV, and bacterial causes. Other causes of esophagitis are irradiation (increases with dose), swallowing corrosive material, and pill-induced.

Pill-induced esophagitis is more likely when pills are taken without water and when the patient is supine. It is especially seen with ASA and NSAIDs, doxycycline, KCl, FeSO4, alendronate (Fosamax©; for postmenopausal osteoporosis; rare), and quinidine. Consider this in a young patient taking medication for acne (doxycycline) with acute onset of odynophagia (painful swallowing).
Treatment for pill-induced esophagitis is to stop the cause of it. For odynophagia with thrush, assume *Candida* and treat with fluconazole. For an immunosuppressed patient with odynophagia and no thrush, treat empirically with fluconazole and, if no response in a few days, workup for other causes.

GE REFLUX DISEASE

Overview

GE Reflux is usually a result of inappropriate transient relaxation of the lower esophageal sphincter (LES). The transient relaxation is, in part, a reflex caused by recently ingested fat in the duodenum. Hiatal hernia is another lesser factor—probably because gastric contents can be trapped in the hiatal pouch [pg 122 #365].
LES pressure is increased by: motilin, acetylcholine, and maybe gastrin. Therefore drugs which increase these mediators tend to decrease reflux. LES pressure is decreased by progesterone (pregnancy increases GE reflux), chocolate, smoking, and some medications, especially those with anticholinergic properties.
Patients with a persistent nonproductive cough, especially with hoarseness, continual clearing of the throat, and a feeling of fullness in the throat should be suspected of having GE reflux disease (GERD). This cough is usually worse at night when the patient is supine.
Most non-cardiac chest pains (70%) are caused by GERD! Most other GI-related chest pains are due to motility disorders. A note: these pains are not necessarily associated with pyrosis (heartburn) or dysphagia.
Extraesophageal manifestations of GERD:
• Nocturnal cough
• Frequent sore throat
• Hoarseness, Laryngitis

notes

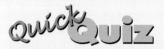
• Loss of dental enamel
• Exacerbation of asthma

This last manifestation notes the very interesting aspect of GERD—its apparent relationship to asthma. Some asthma patients, even without symptoms of GERD, have improvement of their asthma symptoms with GERD treatment. When working up GERD, always ask about asthma symptoms—especially at night.

Complications: esophageal ulcers, stricture, bleeding, and Barrett esophagus (discussed next).

Diagnosis of GERD

If the patient has only the classic symptom of heartburn, the diagnostic workup starts with a therapeutic trial—endoscopy is indicated only if this trial fails. (See Figure 1-1).

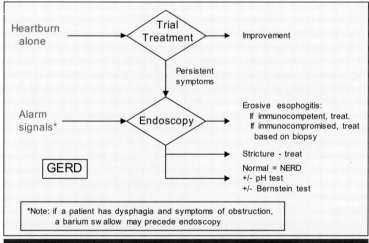

Figure 1-1: Workup of GERD

Alarm signals—indicating the need to endoscope the GERD patient:
• nausea/emesis   • dysphagia
• blood in the stool   • family Hx of PUD
• weight loss   • anorexia
• anemia
• suggestive physical exam
• noncardiac chest pain,
• long duration of frequent symptoms especially in Caucasian males > 45 years old, and
• failure to respond to conventional therapy

If the patient has obstructive symptoms, a barium esophagram may be done before endoscopy. Endoscopy is generally not indicated in GERD patients as only 2% of patients with symptoms of GERD have endoscopic evidence of esophagitis.

Note that 62% of patients with GERD symptoms have a normal esophagus. This is termed nonerosive esophagitis or NERD(!).

The 24-hour intraesophageal pH monitor is indicated for atypical cases such as

1) a patient with refractory symptoms and a normal EGD,

2) a patient with hoarseness, coughing, or atypical chest pain but no classic symptoms of GERD and

3) failure to respond to PPIs.

The pH monitor is similar to a Holter monitor in that the patient keeps a diary of symptoms. The diary logs and pH monitor results are then analyzed for correlation.

A Bernstein test is occasionally used for atypical chest pain; a positive test result is reproduction of symptoms when 0.1 molar HCl is infused into the esophageal lumen.

Treatment of GERD

Treatment of mild to moderate GERD:

First: Head of bed up, weight loss of > 10 lb if overweight or recent weight gain, small meals, no fatty meals in the evening, eat dinner at least 3 hours before bedtime, no sweets at bedtime, stop smoking, and antacids prn. Avoid acidic beverages (e.g., colas, orange juice, wine).

Then try antisecretory drugs: H2 receptor antagonists given BID (vs. daily for PUD). Proton pump inhibitors (PPI) such as omeprazole may be substituted and are often required. Although long-term effects of omeprazole are not known, so far it has been safe. Overall healing of patients with endoscopic evidence of esophagitis (not necessarily GERD!) are: placebo: 25%, H2 blockers and prokinetic drugs: 50%, and proton pump inhibitors: 80%.

The prokinetic drugs, such as metoclopramide (Reglan®), have many side effects with prolonged use. Prokinetic drugs and H2 receptor antagonists are equally effective. Prokinetic drugs do not heal erosive esophagitis (as do all the antisecretory drugs) and are considered adjunctive therapy for GERD after PPIs.

Treatment of severe GERD (i.e., grade 2 or worse esophagitis) requires proton pump inhibitors such as omeprazole and this is continued INDEFINITELY unless the patient has corrective surgery.

notes

Be aware of H^+ rebound if PPIs are stopped abruptly after several months. Also know that PPI treatment leads to parietal cell hyperplasia.

Antireflux surgery (fundoplication; now laparoscopic) should be considered in patients with severe GERD as it has a reasonable success rate. Indications are patients refractory to medical treatment, young patients with severe disease, and as an alternative to long term PPI. With Nissen fundoplication, the lower esophagus is wrapped in a sleeve of the stomach. Side effects of this surgery are bloating, dysphagia, and an inability to belch. A motility study must be done prior to antireflux surgery—if motility is minimal, surgery is contraindicated as you will only cause an iatrogenic dysphagia.

Treat peptic strictures with bougienage. Note that metoclopramide (due to too many side effects) and sucralfate (not very effective) have little use in treatment of GE reflux.

Maintenance therapy may consist of PPIs such as omeprazole (moderate to severe). The H2 receptor blockers are usually ineffective long-term.

Be aware that patients with GERD-related cough/hoarseness require much longer treatment for symptomatic improvement than those with run-of-the-mill heartburn.

BARRETT ESOPHAGUS

Barrett esophagus is a change in cell type—metaplasia—from esophageal squamous to intestinal columnar—caused by chronic GE reflux. 10 to 20% of patients endoscoped for chronic reflux have it! Roughly, patients > 40 years old with a > 10 year history of reflux symptoms (duration is more important than severity) should be endoscoped for evidence of Barrett esophagus. It is especially seen in white males.

Barrett esophagus is associated only with adenocarcinoma (not squamous). Incidence of adenocarcinoma in patients with Barrett esophagus is 30 times normal but, because occurrence of esophageal adenocarcinoma is so low in the normal population, if (at diagnosis) a patient with Barrett esophagus does not have cancer, then life expectancy is normal. Probability of adenocarcinoma is related to the length of Barrett esophagus, presence of a hiatal hernia, degree of dysplasia, and concurrent smoking. With less than 8 cm of Barrett esophagus there is very little chance of progression to dysplasia. Risk of adenocarcinoma is 0.4% per year in patients with Barrett esophagus. Neither antireflux medication nor surgery reverse the epithelial changes of Barrett esophagus.

Endoscopy with biopsy is done every 2-3 years for Barrett esophagus without dysplasia and every 3-6 months for low grade dysplasia. Esophageal resection surgery is indicated for high grade dysplasia. Laser and photodynamic therapy are on the treatment horizon.

ESOPHAGEAL CANCER

Squamous cell cancer of the esophagus comprises about 50% of esophageal cancer and it usually occurs in the proximal 2/3 of the esophagus! Squamous cancer of the esophagus is caused by smoking, alcohol (especially hard liquor),
achalasia, lye stricture, Plummer-Vinson syndrome (see above), and other cancers of the head and neck. Smoking and alcohol have a synergistic carcinogenic effect on the esophagus. Incidence of squamous cancer has a marked geographic variation and its occurrence appears strongly associated with diet and environment.

The other 50% is adenocarcinoma—which has been on the rise (Barrett)—it occurs in the distal 1/3 of the esophagus. See previous section.

If small and localized, do surgical resection. If large or metastasized, treat with combination chemotherapy (cisplatin + 5-FU) plus radiation. This results in a 2 year survival of 38% vs. 10% with radiation alone.

ZENKER DIVERTICULUM

Zenker diverticulum is an outpouching of the upper esophagus. Patients have foul smelling breath and may regurgitate food eaten several days earlier. This is also the most common cause of transfer dysphagia (trouble initiating swallowing) for solid foods but it can also cause transport dysphagia.

Note: Know the indications for EGD, ERCP, pH monitor, and motility studies!

STOMACH
NORMAL PHYSIOLOGY

First a quick review of normal stomach physiology as it relates to gastritis and PUD (See Figure 1-2): G-cells are in the pyloric antrum. Stimulation by food breakdown products such as amino acids causes the G-cells to release gastrin which, like acetylcholine (ACh) and histamine, interacts with specific receptors on the parietal cells in the fundus—stimulating them to produce (via the proton pump) gastric acid. Note that the proton pump is the final common pathway for the action of these three receptors and this is why the proton pump inhibitors such as omeprazole are the strongest anti-gastric acid drugs.

Gastrin is released into the circulation and is therefore an endocrine stimulus for gastric acid release. Gastrin is the dominant mediator of postprandial gastric acid production. ACh, via the vagus nerve, has a direct neurocrine effect while the histamine has a local paracrine effect. Endocrine, neurocrine, paracrine.

Secretin is a negative feedback mediator. Produced in the duodenum in response to the acidified output of the stomach, it both decreases the gastrin production and stimulates output of bicarbonate from the pancreas. A stomach pH < 3 also inhibits gastrin production. This is probably via somatostatin produced by antral D cells. Again, two inhibitors of gastrin secretion are low pH (via somatostatin) and secretin. Note that, in patients with achlorhydria (as in autoimmune gastritis below) or pernicious anemia, the serum gastrin level skyrockets because of the loss of this inhibitory effect.

notes

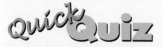

Both gastric acid and pepsin (made from pepsinogen in the presence of acid), in addition to digesting food, attack the mucosal defenses.

Things to know about the mechanical actions of mixing and grinding: 1) this is best studied with a gastric emptying scan. 2) Only particles < 1 mm can pass the pylorus. 3) Peristalsis is activated by a pacemaker.

DYSPEPSIA

Dyspepsia. Most is functional or caused by medications (Fe, ASA, NSAIDs, etc.), but if it is of recent onset and the patient's age is > 40 years, it is anatomic until proven otherwise. Anatomic causes include PUD, gastritis, GERD, cholecystitis, gastroparesis, pancreatitis, cancer, etc. EGD is usually normal. Dyspepsia is generally classified by symptoms as: GERD-like, ulcer-like (improves on antiulcer therapy), and dysmotility-type (improves on promotility drugs such as metoclopramide and erythromycin). There can also be overlaps in the types. "Non-ulcer dyspepsia" is the term defined by a normal EGD.

EROSIVE GASTRITIS

Erosive gastritis (which is frequently hemorrhagic) is due to NSAIDs, alcohol, and severe physiologic stress. Onset in the ICU suggests stress related mucosal damage (SRMD), which is due to severe physiologic stress such as that induced by major surgery or burns. Being on a ventilator or having a coagulopathy are also major risk factors. Just about anything works to prevent SRMD: H2 receptor antagonists, antacids, sucralfate, and even early feedings decrease the incidence of erosive gastritis. Continuous infusion of H2 receptor antagonists is very effective treatment for SRMD. Although it was thought that the decreased acidity in the stomach allow colonization and increase the risk of aspiration pneumonia, it has been shown that there is no increase in aspiration pneumonia with the use of H2 blockers.

CHRONIC GASTRITIS

Chronic (non-erosive) gastritis—two types (A&B).

Type A: Autoimmune, Atrophic, pernicious Anemia, Achlorhydria. It affects the proximal stomach—fundus and body only ("Antrum" is not one of the A words). Autoantibodies against both intrinsic factor and the parietal cells cause a progression to pernicious anemia and to achlorhydria with secondary hypergastrinemia (levels often > 1000 pg/ml). There is no association of cancer with chronic atrophic gastritis itself although there is a 3xN increase in gastric adenocarcinoma with pernicious anemia. Even so, since the incidence of gastric cancer is so low, the diagnosis of pernicious anemia is not enough to warrant periodic endoscopic exams.

Type B is the most common form of gastritis (80%) and, it turns out, is a curable infectious disease! *Helicobacter pylori* is the cause. Virtually all people in third world countries are infected with *H. pylori*. In the U. S., the incidence is about 50% in older patients and 30% overall. Virtually all those infected have a chronic distal/antral gastritis although only a minority have symptoms, and only the symptomatic ones are treated. See PUD below for more on *H. pylori*. Successful treatment of the infection results in resolution of gastritis symptoms in most patients. Again: A patient with chronic distal (antral) gastritis virtually always has *H. pylori* and, when it is eliminated, gastritis usually resolves—although patients may still have dyspepsia.

The gold standard for *H. pylori* testing is histologic examination of biopsied antral mucosa—which is rarely done. The noninvasive tests consist of serologic tests and urease tests.

THE STOMACH

Cardiac zone
Mucous cells
Fundus
Parietal cells
ACh (+)
Histamine (+) (+)
PPIs
(-)
PROTON PUMP
Gastric acid
Duodenum
Pyloric Antrum
Low pH (+)
(-) G-cells
(-) D-cells
Somatostatin
Secretin
Gastrin
Stimulates pancreas

Note: low pH decreases gastrin by stimulating the D-cells to produce somatostatin and the duodenum to produce secretin.

Figure 1-2: Stomach Physiology

notes

Serologic tests (ELISA—IgG) are inexpensive office tests which are very sensitive and specific but only indicate past exposure and are unable to determine active disease—so are not good for checking effectiveness of treatment. On the other hand, a negative *H. pylori* blood test in a dyspeptic patient rules out *H. pylori* as the cause.

Urease tests do check for active disease and are also sensitive (95%) and specific (95%). In one (the CLOtest), the sample is placed on medium containing urea. The ammonia then produced causes an increase in pH, which changes the color of the medium. Breath tests, which use radiolabeled urea, are equally effective. Urease tests are less sensitive if the patient is on a drug which partially suppresses *H. pylori*, such as omeprazole. Cultures are specific but not sensitive.

PEPTIC ULCER
OVERVIEW

Peptic ulcers have 4 well confirmed causes.

1) *Helicobacter pylori* is by far the most common cause of peptic ulcer disease—especially duodenal ulcer disease (70-75%). Lifetime ulcer risk for a person with *H. pylori* infection is 10-15% (higher for men than women). If *H. pylori* can be eradicated, ulcers virtually never recur and the *H. pylori* recurrence rate is very small. The trouble is getting rid of it! If the ulcer does recur, suspect NSAIDs.

2) NSAIDs. The prevalence of ulcers in patients on NSAIDs is 10-30% (!) although many are < 5 mm and do not cause symptoms. NSAIDs cause both gastric and duodenal ulcers—usually gastric (only 5-7% of duodenal ulcers). If NSAIDs are required and the patient is having or has had trouble:
- use COX-2 NSAID (see below)
- use enteric coated NSAIDs;
- use a nonacetylated NSAID (e.g., salsalate = Disalcid®);
- use NSAIDs which are nonacidic pro-drugs (e.g., nabumetone = Relafen®);
- co-administer the NSAID with a prostaglandin E analogue (e.g., misoprostol = Cytotec®) or a PPI. PPIs such as misoprostol are superior to H2 blockers and to sucralfate in the prevention of NSAID-induced ulcers.

Risk factors for conventional NSAID-induced PUD include: 1st 3 months of use, high doses, elderly patient, history of ulcer disease, cardiac disease, concurrent steroids, and serious illness.

Risk of bleeding with conventional NSAIDs:
- General population: 1%. In those using ASA as preventive medicine = 1.5%.
- Female; > 60; or history of PUD/UGI bleed: 3%
- Above 3+ cardiac disease: 9%

Risk of bleeding with COX-2 NSAIDs:
- General population: 0.5%. In those using ASA as preventive medicine = 1%.

COX-2 NSAIDs block the action of cyclooxygenase (COX)—an enzyme which converts arachidonic acid to prostaglandin. COX-1 is the constitutive enzyme while COX-2 is inducible.

COX-1 produces protective prostaglandins in the stomach whereas the inducible COX-2 is involved in inflammatory response. There is a newer NSAID class which is selective for COX-2 (rofecoxib—Vioxx®, celecoxib—Celebrex®, and meloxicam—Mobic®). These COX-2 inhibitor NSAIDs have greatly decreased GI side effects compared to conventional non-selective NSAIDs while retaining the antiinflammatory and pain relief effects. The COX-2 inhibitors are extremely exciting and represent a leap forward in our understanding of the inflammatory process. They are being evaluated in areas such as the prevention of colon cancer, decreasing adenomatous polyps in familial polyposis syndrome, Bartter syndrome (salt-wasting), and Alzheimer disease—where use/dosage of conventional NSAIDs has been limited by GI side effects.

3) High acid secreting states such as Zollinger-Ellison (3-5% of duodenal ulcers).

4) Crohn disease of the duodenum/stomach.

What about tobacco? In both gastric and duodenal ulcer disease, smoking exacerbates the ulcer. For those not caused by *H. pylori*, smoking also decreases the healing rate and increases recurrence and perforation rate. Commonly these recurrences are asymptomatic.

Previously, the incidence of PUD was higher in men than women but now the male to female ratio is approaching 1. Type of diet, personality, and occupation are not significant etiologic factors! Weight loss is uncommon in PUD. Notes: alcohol is not ulcerogenic! Corticosteroids alone are not ulcerogenic but they double the risk of serious NSAID-associated gastrointestinal complication—risk of bleeding may be 10x!

DIAGNOSIS of PUD

If a non-perforated ulcer is suspected, EGD is the diagnostic procedure of choice. UGI is less sensitive than the EGD. If an ulcer is found, serum gastrin levels may be indicated (specifics discussed under the type of ulcer). The presence of *H. pylori* is diagnosed as described in the gastritis section above.

Perforated gastric and duodenal ulcers often cause free air in the peritoneal space which can be seen on an upright abdominal x-ray. If a perforated ulcer is suspected, do the upright x-ray first!...EGD and UGI are contraindicated. Also know that absence of an ulcer crater means there is no risk of hemorrhage, perforation, or scarring!

Know that the pain of an ulcer tends to be gnawing whereas that of a perforated ulcer is usually severe.

notes

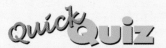

1) What is the most common cause of peptic ulcer disease?

2) True or False: Type of diet, personality, and occupation are significant factors in the development of peptic ulcer disease.

3) What is a good drug for PUD in renal insufficiency patients? Why?

4) Are corticosteroids used as sole therapy ulcerogenic?

5) Do corticosteroids accentuate the bleeding effect of NSAIDs in PUD?

TREATMENT of PUD

Treatment of PUD targets combinations of 3 main factors:
1) *H. pylori* treatment.
2) Stop acid secretion (H2 receptor antagonists, PPIs).
3) Stop exacerbating processes (smoking, taking NSAIDs).
Two other factors, mucosal protection (sucralfate) and acid neutralization with antacids, are used less frequently.

Treat any *H. pylori* infection associated with PUD. General aspects of therapy:
1) Treat for 10-14 days. One week is insufficient.
2) Usually triple drug therapy is used—two antibiotics and a proton pump inhibitor. A good one with an eradication rate of about 85% is O-CLAM (omeprazole 20mg + clarithromycin 500mg + amoxicillin 1g—bid x 10d). Recurrence rate is very low.
Know that the more drugs the better! Single and dual drug therapies are ineffective.
Note that *H. pylori* develops resistance to metronidazole and to clarithromycin when used alone—so any recent use of these antibiotics precludes their use. Also regimens that include metronidazole are less effective in the U.S. than Europe—probably because there is increased resistance to metronidazole in the US.

If the patient tests negative for *H. pylori* infection and exacerbating factors such as NSAIDs have been addressed, antisecretory drugs and antacids can be used. Sucralfate is effective in the treatment of non-*H. pylori* PUD but its qid dosage is a hassle and PPIs are better. Sucralfate binds to the ulcer site where it adsorbs bile salts and forms a barrier to prevent acid penetration. Sucralfate is often the drug of choice in renal patients because it also binds PO4.
Stop smoking—it increases risk of recurrence and perforation in ulcers not associated with *H. pylori* or untreated *H. pylori* ulcers.
Indications for surgery in PUD:
  UGI bleed—active bleed unable to stop via endoscopic therapy. Surgery is only required in 5% of UGI bleeds.
  Gastric outlet obstruction—initial treatment is balloon dilation. Surgery required in ~25%.
  Recurrent/refractory ulcers (rare)
  Perforation—laparoscopic repair may be possible.
  ZES.

NOTES: DUODENAL vs. GASTRIC ULCER

Duodenal ulcer. Again, 50-75% are due to *H. pylori*. 10-25% NSAIDs, and 1-3% increased acid secretion (ZES). Duodenal ulcers have a closer association with acid hypersecretion than gastric ulcers (not enough bicarbonate in the duodenum to neutralize all the acid) [pg 126, #376-380].

Gastric ulcers [pg 124, #371 & 372] not associated with *H. pylori* are treated for 3 months because these heal more slowly than duodenal ulcers. Misoprostol, a synthetic prostaglandin, and PPIs are superior to H2 blockers and sucralfate in the prevention of NSAID-induced ulcers.

Although gastric ulcers have previously been thought to be associated with gastric cancer, studies have not shown this to be true! On the other hand, all nonhealing gastric ulcers should be examined via endoscopy and have a cytologic exam of at least six biopsy samples to rule out gastric cancer. Achlorhydria after stimulation with a meal virtually never occurs in a patient with a benign gastric ulcer.

BLEEDING ULCERS

Bleeding ulcers. Risk factors for bleeding include use of NSAIDs. The bleeding risk is dose-related. As mentioned previously, corticosteroids are not ulcerogenic alone, but they may increase the NSAID-associated bleeding 10 fold!
Risk factors indicating a severe bleed and/or a high risk of further rebleed include
  • hemodynamic instability,
  • recurrent red-colored hematemesis or hematochezia, and
  • lack of clearing of gastric lavage effluent. On endoscopy,
  • the size of the ulcer and
  • visible vessels on a nonbleeding ulcer increase the risk for rebleed.
Endoscopy is the diagnostic procedure of choice for UGI bleed. It should be done emergently if the patient has any of the first 3 just-mentioned findings.

Medical therapy: Gastric lavage does not stop bleeding or prevent rebleeding. Vasoconstrictors also are ineffective. Decreasing gastric acidity does not prevent rebleeding but is appropriate as treatment to heal the ulcer. Orally administered medication is effective, therefore an intravenous H2 receptor antagonist is usually not indicated unless the patient must remain NPO.
Endoscopic therapy. The following are equally effective: bipolar electrocoagulation, heater-probe therapy, and injection therapy. Surgery is done if endoscopic therapy fails; angiographic therapy is considered only if the patient is not a candidate for surgery.

notes

Note: IV and PO PPIs after endoscopic therapy for bleeding ulcer decreases:
1) recurrent bleeding
2) mortality
3) need for surgery

PPIs protect the clot by increasing intragastric pH > 6.0.

ZOLLINGER-ELLISON

Zollinger-Ellison syndrome (ZES) occurs when a gastrinoma, which produces gastrin continuously, causes refractory (usually duodenal bulb and stomach) ulcers and diarrhea +/- steatorrhea. The diarrhea/steatorrhea is from malabsorption caused by acidification of duodenal contents. Gastrinomas most frequently occur in the duodenum (~50%) or pancreas (~25%), less frequently in the stomach, lymph nodes, and spleen. 90% are found in what is called the "ZE triangle"—which includes the porta hepatis, mid-duodenum, and the head of the pancreas. 80% are of the sporadic form; 20% are associated with MEN type 1. Remember: other conditions associated with an elevated gastrin level are pernicious anemia, vitiligo, chronic gastritis, renal failure, and hyperthyroidism. Also remember that gastric carcinoids can be caused by long-standing hypergastrinemic states.

Treatment: All newly diagnosed ZE patients without evidence of metastatic disease warrant surgical exploration. 1/3 will be cured by resection of the primary tumor. Even with metastatic disease, ZES is usually treated aggressively, often with resection if the primary tumor, because the mass effect of the tumor tissue can eventually cause problems. A PPI is now the drug of choice for medical treatment of ZES.

CARCINOID

Gastric carcinoid is usually a result of a chronic hypergastrinemic states such as that seen in ZES and autoimmune gastritis/pernicious anemia—both of which are discussed previously. It may also be associated with vitiligo! Gastrin is trophic to the enterochromaffin type cells of the stomach, leading to hyperplasia and occasionally to gastric carcinoids. Note that the proton pump inhibitor omeprazole has not been shown to cause carcinoids (10 years worth of data). Carcinoids often cause alcohol intolerance and facial flushing and may lead to niacin deficiency. Also see pg 1-15 for more on carcinoids under Chronic Diarrhea.

GASTRIC CANCER

Gastric cancer [pg 125, #373-375]. There are two distinct forms of gastric cancer; a proximal diffuse type and a distal intestinal type. The incidence of distal gastric cancer had been decreasing until about 20 years ago; since then its incidence has been holding steady. The proximal type has been steadily increasing. Either type is usually an adenocarcinoma (90%).

It appears that distal gastric cancer is most strongly associated with environmental factors and the increased risk is pretty much irreversibly set early in life. A summary of risk factors:
• A diet low in fruits and vegetables and high in dried, smoked, and salted foods
• Foods rich in nitrates (animal studies)
• Genetic factors (family history, blood type A)
• Atrophic gastritis and pernicious anemia
• *H. pylori* infection (independent of ulcer disease!)
• Other: Barrett esophagus, distal gastrectomy, uranium mining, inversely related to socioeconomic status.

Neither alcohol consumption nor gastric ulcers have been proven to cause gastric cancer—as previously alleged —even though gastric cancer appears as an ulcer.

Diagnosis of gastric cancer. Often an ulcer is picked up on barium contrast study (double contrast is better). If it appears benign, it can be treated; endoscopy and biopsy need be done only if it does not heal. Endoscopy with multiple biopsies is the diagnostic procedure of choice. Tumor markers, such as carcinoembryonic antigen (CEA) and alpha fetoprotein (AFP), are of no use as early markers for gastric cancer.

Prognosis is determined by stage (TNM classification). Because it is largely asymptomatic until advanced, <10% are found in the early gastric cancer stage (confined to the mucosa and submucosa, T1N0M0). 5 year survival rate varies from 50% for treated stage I to 3% for stage IV. Survival rates are much higher in Japan—90% (I) and 9% (IV)!!—which may be due to their more aggressive treatment, difference in rates of the proximal vs. distal cancers, or difference in staging (more lymph nodes are removed in Japan so spread to nodes is more likely to be picked up).

Treatment consists of surgical removal of the cancer and adjacent lymph nodes. Adjuvant combination chemotherapy prolongs survival. Adjuvant radiotherapy is investigational.

OTHER GASTRIC SYNDROMES

Dumping syndrome consists of postprandial vasomotor symptoms: palpitations, sweating, light-headedness. There are two types. The early type occurs 30 minutes after eating and is of uncertain etiology. The late type occurs 90 minutes or more after eating and is probably due to hypoglycemia. Both types are treated identically with restriction of sweets and lactose-containing foods, and frequent small meals.

Post-gastrectomy syndromes include not only the above-described dumping syndrome and reflux gastritis but also afferent loop syndrome and blind loop syndrome. Afferent loop syndrome presents with abdominal bloating and pain 20 minutes to 1 hour after eating; symptoms are often relieved by vomiting. The emesis is often bile-colored. It is thought to be caused by an incompletely draining afferent loop which fills with biliary and pancreatic secretions. Blind loop syndrome is bacterial overgrowth in a loop (in this case, afferent loop) manifested by fat and B12 malabsorption.

Delayed gastric emptying (gastroparesis) is seen in diabetics and in patients after a vagotomy. These patients have a pre-

notes

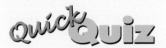

Quick Quiz

1) What is the usual cause of carcinoid?
2) Carcinoid may be associated with which skin condition?
3) How do you rule out gastric cancer in a patient with a nonhealing gastric ulcer?
4) Most gastric carcinomas are of what type?
5) Does alcohol cause gastric cancer?
6) When are barium enemas contraindicated in IBD?
7) Sulfasalazine is ineffective in which types of CD?
8) What are the side effects of sulfasalazine?
9) What drugs decrease the relapse rate in CD? In UC?

disposition to bezoars and reflux gastritis. Diagnose this with a radioisotope labeled solid meal. Treat it with metoclopramide or erythromycin as a liquid suspension 125-250 mg T.I.D. before meals.

Note that oral ketoconazole requires gastric acidity to be effective. If there is achlorhydria, either give the ketoconazole with acid or give oral fluconazole, which is similar but not affected by low gastric acid. Note that 50% of AIDS patients have decreased stomach acid and are therefore especially prone to ketoconazole failure.

INTESTINES

INFLAMMATORY BOWEL DISEASE

Common Factors

Inflammatory Bowel Disease (IBD)—Crohn disease (CD) and ulcerative colitis (UC)—in both types, the patient's family members are at increased risk of IBD and the patient has an increased risk of GI cancer—but the risk of cancer is much higher in long-standing UC than in CD. Toxic megacolon is a complication in both, so a barium enema is contraindicated in both types if the patient is thought to be having an acute exacerbation of UC or CD. Infectious colitis, early CD, and UC all can appear identically on sigmoidoscopy. Stool examination for WBCs, O&P, C&S, and *C. difficile* toxin assay are part of the initial workup. Refer to Table 1-1 as you review CD and UC.

Smoking is associated with both CD and UC but not in the way you might think. Smokers are more likely than the normal population to develop CD, while UC often exacerbates after someone stops smoking!

Remember that the incidence of IBD is 1/20th the incidence of colon cancer! It is rare. Most bloody diarrhea is not due to IBD.

The main drugs used to treat IBD include sulfasalazine, 5-aminosalicylate preparations, olsalazine, prednisone, metronidazole, and azathioprine and its metabolite, 6-mercaptopurine. Also methotrexate, cyclosporine, and monoclonal antibodies to TNF-α.

Sulfasalazine is split, by bacterial action in the colon, into sulfapyridine and mesalamine (5-amino salicylic acid). Mesalamine is the active component of sulfasalazine—hence sulfasalazine is ineffective for CD of the small bowel. The other breakdown product, sulfapyridine, is absorbed in the colon, acetylated in the liver, and excreted in the urine. Sulfapyridine is a highly reactive sulfa moiety which is responsible for most of the side effects of sulfasalazine such as reversible infertility in men, leukopenia, and headache.

Mesalamine (5-aminosalicylic acid) is rapidly absorbed from the upper digestive tract and therefore it is used orally only for small bowel involvement. For colon disease it is either given rectally—either as an enema or suppository—or in a formulation designed to delay absorption of mesalamine. One interesting formulation is olsalazine which is an aminosalicylic acid dimer which requires colonic azo-reduction (as does sulfasalazine) to reduce into two molecules of aminosalicylate in the colon.

Metronidazole is used for perianal abscesses and fistulas in CD and for peritonitis in UC. Combined with a 5-ASA analog, it is useful as maintenance therapy for CD.

6-mercaptopurine and azathioprine (which metabolizes to 6-MP) are prednisone sparing drugs useful in both Crohn and UC; it usually takes 3-4 months to show an effect with these. Also, because these two drugs have bone marrow suppressive effects, CBC should be monitored monthly. There is no report of increased malignancy with long term use of either one. The drugs that decrease the relapse rate in CD are azathioprine, 6-mercaptopurine, and mesalamine while ALL the standard drugs decrease the relapse rate in UC!

Use in pregnancy:

FDA risk category B: Metronidazole, prednisone, and sulfasalazine (and probably its derivatives 5-ASA and olsalazine—but these have not been given an FDA risk category yet).

6-MP and azathioprine are risk category D. Don't use!

Crohn Disease

Overview

Crohn disease (CD; regional enteritis) [pg 129, #385-387]. Although most patients present with this disease in their 20-30's, the disease can present at any age and there is even a second smaller peak of incidence in the 70-80 year-olds. The incidence of CD is increasing. There is only a slightly increased risk of GI cancer with CD; long-term CD patients may be screened every other year for cancer.

CD is more indolent than UC. Because of this, it is less responsive to treatment and it is harder to get these patients off steroids. Patients with CD are more likely to have perianal fistulae and abscesses. They are also more likely to have strictures, inflammatory masses, and associated obstruction. One big problem with CD is the high rate of recurrence. It was once thought to be 50% at 10 years but this is the symptomatic recurrence rate. Radiologic/endoscopic recurrence rate is 75% at 3 years (!)—and only 50% are symptomatic.

notes

Diagnosis

Diagnosis of CD is made by finding patchy, focal, and aphthous ulcers and deep transmural ulcers (called "Crohn's craters") with occasional strictures and fistula formation. Granulomas seen on a biopsy specimen are pathognomonic but infrequently seen. A tetrad to remember for "Crohn's colitis" is rectal sparing, skip lesions, perirectal disease, and contiguous ileocolic disease. These patients may get fever, abdominal pain, and systemic symptoms. One classic but uncommon feature of CD is the string sign which may be seen in the terminal ileum during a small bowel follow-through. The terminal ileum is so edematous and/or fibrotic that the lumen is compressed and shows up as a string of contrast. The edema pushes the rest of the bowel away so the "string" shows up well. If this narrowing of the lumen is seen elsewhere in the colon, it is called an apple-core lesion (which suggests cancer). Bowel involvement in CD: 30% colon only, 40% small bowel only, 30% both.

Note that problems related to disease/resection of the terminal ileum are found in CD—but not in UC. These problems include calcium oxalate kidney stones, cholesterol gallstones, B12 deficiency, hypocalcemia (vitamin D malabsorption), bile acid-induced diarrhea, and malabsorption.

Terminal Ileum Problems

Bile acid induced diarrhea is usually the cause of diarrhea in Crohn patients when less than 100 cm of distal ileum is resected. It is due to bile acid stimulation of salt and H_2O secretion by the colon and is treated with bile acid sequestrants (e.g., cholestyramine), which bind and inactivate the bile acids. When more than 100 cm of distal ileum is resected, the patient gets steatorrhea from greatly decreased bile acids (synthesis does not keep up with GI loss without the distal ileum resorption). These patients are treated with a low-fat diet in addition to the bile acid sequestrants. They may infrequently be given supplemental medium-chain triglycerides.

Treatment Overview

Medical treatment of CD utilizes sulfasalazine, 5-amino salicylate, olsalazine, prednisone, metronidazole, azathioprine and its metabolite, 6-mercaptopurine, and infliximab (Remicade®). (See Table 1-2.) KNOW!:

- Prednisone is more effective in UC than CD— again probably due to the indolent nature of CD. In CD, prednisone is more effective than sulfasalazine when CD affects only the small intestine.
- Infliximab (Remicade®) is an IgG monoclonal antibody to tumor necrosis factor α (TNF-α) which is helpful in patients refractory to corticosteroids and especially in patients with fistulas without high grade obstruction. It also facilitates withdrawal from corticosteroids.

- Metronidazole is effective especially for fistulas and perianal CD (only used for UC when there is fulminant disease with peritonitis). Combined with a 5-ASA analog, it is useful as maintenance therapy for CD.
- 6-mercaptopurine (6-MP) and azathioprine are used with Crohn patients who can not be weaned off prednisone. Note: long-term treatment with 6-MP and with azathioprine have been shown to decrease recurrence rates in CD.

Like 6-MP and azathioprine, mesalamine and olsalazine also probably decrease the relapse rate in CD. Prednisone and metronidazole do not affect relapse rate.

Surgery & Recurrence

Surgery is only for intractable disease and specific serious complications. 60% of Crohn patients undergo surgery in the first 5 years! They require surgery again after about eight years. Hopefully these numbers will prove to decrease with medical therapy (esp. 6-MP, infliximab). The incidence of recurrence after surgery depends on
1) the site—ileocolic is highest—and
2) nature of the complication—obstruction, perforation, and abscess have higher incidence and rates of recurrence.

Essentially, the worse the disease where you cut, the more likely the recurrence at the surgical site. The best results are obtained with colectomy and ileostomy for Crohn colitis when there is no ileal inflammation (> 60% have no remission!).

Treatment scenarios for CD:

Colon only: Sulfasalazine, mesalamine enemas, or olsalazine. Sulfasalazine is about $25/mo vs. $200-300/mo for mesalamine, et. al.. So sulfasalazine is the first choice—then 5-ASA drugs if required because of intolerance to the side effects of sulfasalazine.

Any ileum or small bowel involvement: mesalamine.

Fistula or perianal: Infliximab by IV infusion; metronidazole;

Table 1-1: Comparison of Crohn Disease and Ulcerative Colitis		
Inflammatory Bowel Disease - Comparisons		
	Crohn Disease	Ulcerative Colitis
Lesions	Focal, skip, deep	Shallow, continuous
Clinical course	Indolent	More acute
Prednisone	Less responsive	Very responsive
Granulomas	Pathognomonic	None
Rectal Involvement	Rectal sparing in 50%	Rectum ALWAYS involved
Perianal disease	Abscesses, fistulas	None
Small Bowel Involvement	> 50%	Backwash ileitis in < 10%

notes

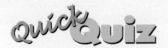

1) What is the significance of an "apple-core" lesion in patients with CD?

2) What is the usual etiology of diarrhea in CD patients with more than 100cm of distal ileum removed? Less than 100cm of distal ileum removed? What is the treatment for each?

3) Review and know the treatment of CD and UC.

4) Which more commonly involves the rectum—CD or UC?

5) What serological marker may be found in 65-75% of patients with UC?

6) Name the skin lesions associated with UC.

ciprofloxacin.

Steroid dependent: 6-MP or azathioprine.

Corticosteroids are a second line drug in this disease. They are used if there is decreased response to the 5-ASA drugs.

Ulcerative Colitis

Overview

Ulcerative colitis (UC) consists of uniform, continuous mucosal inflammation with shallow ulcers extending proximally from the rectum [pg 130, #388-390]. There is usually a sharp margin between the area of involvement and the normal mucosa. The area of involvement tends to remain the same from the time of diagnosis but does extend more proximally in 10%.

65-75% of UC patients are P-ANCA positive. This is of little use clinically (low sensitivity & specificity).

The main symptoms of UC are abdominal pain and bloody diarrhea. Clinical course and degree of involvement are variable—from mild ulcerative proctitis (rectal area only) with minimal symptoms to severe colitis of the entire colon with bad cramps, liquid stools with blood and pus, anemia, extraintestinal manifestations (below), and constitutional symptoms. Tenesmus and constipation may be the major symptoms with ulcerative proctitis.

Extraintestinal Manifestations

Extraintestinal manifestations of UC include: RF negative arthritis, skin lesions (E. nodosum and pyoderma gangrenosum), iritis/episcleritis/uveitis, venous thrombosis, ankylosing spondylitis, pericholangitis, and sclerosing cholangitis. The skin lesions correlate with disease activity. Primary sclerosing cholangitis is also associated with HLA-B8, and ankylosing spondylitis and uveitis are associated with HLA-B27. The complications associated with HLA antigens tend not to improve with improvement of the colitis whereas the other problems mentioned here usually do get better! Extraintestinal manifestations of IBD are usually seen in IBD patients with colitis (so they are usually associated with UC, although they can be seen in CD involving the colon).

"JSEM" is the mnemonic for diseases seen with colonic disease (colitis): **J**oint, **S**kin, **E**yes, **M**outh.

You must rule out the infectious causes of colitis: *E. coli* O157:H7, *Shigella*, *Salmonella*, *Yersinia*, *Campylobacter*, *C. difficile*, and amebiasis. Especially *Campylobacter*—as it can have a chronic, relapsing course that mimics UC. *C. difficile*

Table 1-2: Treatment of Inflammatory Bowel Disease. Comparison of treatments used in ulcerative colits and Crohn Disease.

TREATMENT OF INFLAMMATORY BOWEL DISEASE						
ULCERATIVE COLITIS						
SEVERITY: ...definition of severity		MILD	MODERATE	SEVERE	FULMINANT	REMISSION
	Stools/d	< 4	Between mild and severe	> 6	> 10	Normal
	KUB	Normal		Air, edema, thumbprinting	Bowel dilatation	
	Physical exam	Normal; but intermittant fecal blood		Fever, Abd tenderness, freq fecal blood	Fever, Abd tenderness and distention	
TREATMENT:		Distal disease: Rectal corticosteroids; oral or rectal aminosalicylates Extensive colon involvement: Oral aminosalicylates		Distal disease: Oral or rectal corticosteroids Extensive colon involvement:	IV corticosteroids IV cyclosporine if resistant to corticosteroids	Oral aminosalicylates (rectal okay if distal disease) Oral azathioprine or mercaptopurine if steroid dependent or refractory.
CROHN DISEASE						
SEVERITY:		MILD	MODERATE	SEVERE/FULMINANT	POSTOP	REMISSION
TREATMENT:		Oral amino-salycilates; Metronidazole	Oral corticosteroids; Azathioprine, 6-MP, or methotrexate if steroid depdt or refractory	IV corticosteroids; IV infliximab; Elemental diet or TPN = transient benefit	Metronidazole (delays anastomotic recurrence - danger of neuropathy)	Oral aminosalicylate; Azathioprine or 6-MP especially if steroid dependent or refractory; Note: 6-MP is now standard maintenence therapy.

Note the differences and similarities in these treatments! Metronidazole and diet (bowel rest) are ineffective in UC. Rectal preparations are only used in UC of the distal colon

notes

is usually thought of as an acute disease but it can be symptomatic for 1-3 months.

LFTs, especially alkaline phosphatase, are checked initially and periodically. If the value becomes 2 x nl and persists, a workup for sclerosing cholangitis is indicated.

Cancer in UC

Risk of cancer in patients with UC is high—0.5%/year and up to 10% in 20 years. Risk is increased with duration and extent of UC—pancolitis has the highest risk whereas ulcerative proctitis has no increased risk. Any patient who has had UC for 10 years should have a colonoscopy with biopsy to check for dysplasia. Once started, normal colonoscopic screening for cancer is every 1-3 years.

UC is cured with surgery. Complete colectomy is recommended for patients with dysplasia in a mass lesion and for high grade dysplasia in flat mucosa. Colonoscopy should be repeated in 6 months if there is low grade dysplasia without inflammation. Repeat in 6-12 months for dysplasia with inflammation (usually not precancerous). There is no increased risk for cancer if there is atrophy without dysplasia.

Other indications for surgery besides cancer considerations are intractable disease, growth retardation in children, perforation, toxicity, and exsanguinating hemorrhage.

Treatment of UC

Medical treatment of UC (know). Therapy is changing due to the advent of 5-ASA compounds without sulfa. Also note the addition of corticosteroids. UC, being a more acute inflammatory process, responds to steroids much better than CD. See Table 1-2.

For mild disease, there are several options. Oral sulfasalazine, oral mesalamine, rectal mesalamine (suppository for proctitis; enema for proctosigmoiditis), and hydrocortisone enemas. All have similar efficacy—75% response and 30% remission after 2 months. The HC enemas have few side-effects and give quicker symptom relief than mesalamine.

For moderate to severe UC, initial therapy is oral prednisone. Patients with fulminant UC should be hospitalized and treated with IV corticosteroids and antibiotics (metronidazole); the patient may need a colectomy if the fulminant symptoms persist for > 24 hours.

Maintenance therapy after remission: sulfasalazine, mesalamine, olsalazine given daily for 1-2 years. Azathioprine and 6-mercaptopurine are used for frequent recurrences/steroid dependence; treatment may take several months to show an effect. Cyclosporine effects short-term remission in 40-50% of patients with severe colitis but long-term in only 20%—limited use

A few buzzwords: Tenesmus (UC); Rectal bleeding (UC); Fecal soiling (think fistula = CD); Hydronephrosis without stones (obstruction from inflammatory mass = CD); Pneumaturia (think fistula to the bladder = CD).

Overview

Diarrhea is defined variably as more than 200-250 gm/day of stool. Average daily output is 150-180 gm.

Classification of diarrhea can be according to 3 mechanisms: osmotic, secretory, and increased motility. First we will compare and contrast osmotic and secretory mechanisms (note that "[x]"means "concentration of x"):

Overview: In all normal bowel contents the number of cations $[Na^+]$ plus $[K^+]$ are equal to the anions: $[Cl^-]$ + $[HCO3-]$ + other absorbable anions (mostly short-chained fatty acids which should be absorbed early in bowel transit). Therefore, calculated stool osmolality can be said to be = $2[Na^+ + K^+]$. Since stool osmolality is equal to serum osmolality, it is generally 290 mOsm/L—more accurately 280-300 mOsm/L but to simplify, I will say 290 throughout this discussion. That stool is isotonic is also true for all types of diarrhea. Because the fluid in secretory diarrhea is, in essence, an ultrafiltrate of the serum, secretory diarrhea is similar to normal stool in that $2[Na^+ + K^+]$ = 290 mOsm/L, whereas in osmotic diarrhea, part of the osmolality is due to unmeasured, nonabsorbable, osmotically active molecules—so the $2[Na^+ + K^+]$ is much less than 290 mOsm/L—this difference is usually > 50 mOsm/L.

Secretory Diarrhea

In secretory diarrhea, $2[Na^+ + K^+]$ of the stool is equal to 290 mOsm/L (i.e., measured serum osmolality). There is more stool volume in secretory diarrhea than in osmotic diarrhea, often > 1 L/d, so there is obviously an increased secretion of electrolytes and the patient is at risk for an electrolyte deficiency. There are many causes of secretory diarrhea:
• enterotoxins from E. coli, Cholera, and S. aureus
• villous adenomas
• gastrinomas
• VIPomas which produce vasoactive intestinal peptide (VIP)
• microscopic colitis
• collagenous colitis
• bile acids
• **irritative** laxatives (e.g., phenolphthalein – not available in US anymore but is widely used elsewhere)

A 24-48 hr hour fast does not stop secretory diarrhea except in fatty acid and bile acid related diarrheas.

See Table 1-3.

Osmotic Diarrhea

In osmotic diarrhea, (serum osmolality - $2[Na^+ + K^+]$) > 50. So there is at least a 50 mOsm/L osmotic gap which is due to a nonabsorbable osmotic agent. A 24 hour fast does resolve the diarrhea. Lactase deficiency is one of the most common causes of osmotic diarrhea. Other common causes are: Mg-containing laxatives and antacids, non- or poorly absorbable carbohydrates (xylitol, lactulose, sorbitol, fructose), and nu-

notes

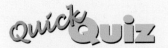

trient malabsorption (pancreatic insufficiency, celiac sprue, bacterial overgrowth...). If an osmotic diarrhea persists despite a 24 hour fast, suspect surreptitious ingestion of a Mg-containing antacid. Most laxatives cause an osmotic diarrhea, including castor oil.

What if the stool osmolality is greater than serum osmolality? This indicates an improper stool collection procedure.

Increased Motility

Increased Motility: The last mechanism is increased motility. The dysmotility syndromes include antibiotic-associated diarrhea, hyperthyroidism, carcinoid, and irritable bowel. Erythromycin is one of the most common causes of antibiotic-associated diarrhea. It binds to motilin receptors thereby increasing bowel motility. This property of erythromycin makes it useful as a treatment for gastroparesis. Treatment for most antibiotic-associated diarrhea is stopping the drug. Antibiotic- associated colitis is a different animal (*C. difficile*) and discussed later.

Different mechanisms of diarrhea may occur together in certain diseases. In celiac disease, osmotic and secretory mecha-

nisms coexist because there is malabsorption of carbohydrates (osmotic) and fat (secretory). Exudative diarrhea (i.e., high fecal WBCs; includes invasive bacteria and inflammatory bowel diseases) contains all three mechanisms: inflammation causes altered motility, malabsorption again can cause both osmotic and secretory components.

DIARRHEA CLASSIFICATION by ACUTE vs. CHRONIC

Overview

Another way of categorizing diarrhea is acute (**I**) vs. chronic (**II**). Acute is < 4 weeks duration. Note that the above osmolal criteria are clinically useful only for chronic diarrhea.

Acute Diarrhea

Introduction

I. Acute diarrhea is usually of an infectious etiology but it may also be caused by food poisoning or drug side-effects.

First we will have a brief overview of the diagnosis and treatment of acute diarrhea—then we will discuss specific organisms.

Diagnosis of acute diarrhea: Do the simple things first! Check diet history. Lab: First check fecal WBC—if elevated, then do C+S, O+P (O+P also if positive travel history), and +/- sigmoidoscopy with biopsy. If *E. coli* O157:H7 is suspected, you need to specifically ask for MacConkey-sorbitol agar for the stool culture media.

Treatment: Generally, invasive diarrhea is treated with TMP/SMX, but use erythromycin for *Campylobacter* and metronidazole for giardiasis and amebiasis. TMP/SMX may prolong *Salmonella* infections which are otherwise usually self-limited. Quinolones (especially ciprofloxacin) are effective in all these except giardiasis and amebiasis and are an alternative first choice. Another big exception is *E. coli* O157:H7 infection which is treated only symptomatically if mild or moderate, with hemodialysis if severe.

Infectious Causes of Acute Diarrhea

Enterotoxigenic vs. Invasive
In both of the following types, agents need to adhere to the bowel wall. Also in both, decreased gastric acid may increase susceptibility.

1. Enterotoxigenic—*Vibrio cholerae* [pg 14, #41], *E. coli* (usual cause of Travelers' diarrhea), and viruses. With enterotoxigenic, the stool C+S usually grows normal flora only. It usually has a large volume, no blood or leukocytes, and no symptoms of systemic infection. Most are treated with antimotility drugs and fluid replacement. Antibiotic treatment is indicated for Travelers' diarrhea if the patient is febrile (TMP/SMX, ciprofloxacin, doxycycline, bismuth-subsalicylate), otherwise usually treat by replacing fluid and antimotility drugs (e.g., diphenoxylate+atropine [Lomotil®]).

Table 1-3: Osmotic vs Secretory Diarrhea		
	OSMOTIC	SECRETORY
Volume /day	< 1 L	> 1 L
Effect of Fasting on diarrhea	Decreases > 50%	Decreases < 20%
Stool Osmolality- mosm/L	290	290
Na⁺ K⁺ Na⁺ + K⁺	40 20 60	105 40 145
2(Na⁺ + K⁺)	120	290
Osmotic gap	> 50	< 50

notes

Enterotoxigenic *E. Coli* is the usual cause of Travelers' diarrhea. These are different from regular *E. Coli* in that they have plasmids which give them both increased adherence and heat-labile enterotoxin. Treatment discussed in the ID booklet.

2. Invasive (a subclass of exudative)—*Campylobacter* (most common!), *Salmonella* (especially suspect this in sickle cell patients and in patients with achlorhydria; may cause joint pains), *Shigella*, *E. coli* O157:H7, *Clostridia*, and *Yersinia* (associated with joint pains, rash, and abdominal pain which may mimic appendicitis or regional enteritis). Occasionally *E. histolytica* (amebiasis), and *Giardia*. And yes, invasive diarrhea does cause histologic damage. Invasive diarrhea typically contains many WBCs +/- blood and the patient is usually febrile. The exception to this is giardiasis in which there are no RBCs or WBCs in the stool specimen.

Incidence of these organisms in diarrheal stool in a recent U.S. study (n = 30,000): Campylobacter 2.3%, Salmonella 1.8%, Shigella 1.1%, E. coli O157:H7 0.4% [Slutsker et al.].

Bacteria

Campylobacter jejuni is usually ingested from undercooked/raw poultry but may also be obtained from drinking water from mountain streams, foreign travel, or contact with infected dogs and cats. 30-50% of all raw chicken in the markets have Campylobacter! Know that Guillain-Barré syndrome is linked to antecedent Campylobacter enteritis in 1/3 of cases. Symptoms of Campylobacter enteritis include abdominal cramping and diarrhea which is often bloody. Symptoms last 5-7 days but may be shortened by taking erythromycin.

Salmonella is especially associated with ingestion of raw eggs or contaminated ice cream. The larger the dose of Salmonella, the worse the disease. Salmonellosis consists of fever, abdominal cramps, and diarrhea—often bloody.

Shigella causes shigellosis which has similar symptoms as salmonellosis. Most disease is transmitted by infected persons or food or water contaminated by infected persons. Only a few organisms can cause disease. Resistance to antibiotics is increasing so it is important to know local resistance patterns.

Outbreaks of *E. coli* O157:H7 food-borne infections are becoming more frequent—especially in the North and Northwest US. The incidence of *E. coli* O157:H7 infection is greater than that of *Shigella*! Dairy cattle appear to be a major reservoir and the disease is linked to eating undercooked beef and unpasteurized milk or apple juice. This strain of *E. coli* produces a verotoxin which may cause bloody diarrhea, hemorrhagic colitis, *hemolytic uremic syndrome* (HUS), and simulate TTP. HUS classically has the triad of kidney failure, thrombocytopenia with purpura, and hemolytic anemia (see Hematology section).

Clostridium difficile causes pseudomembranous colitis ("antibiotic associated colitis"). This usually presents about a week after starting antibiotics but it may start up to 6-8 weeks after antibiotics are stopped! With this disease, the bowel has a hyperemic mucosa with plaque-like lesions and a pseudomembrane [pg 131, #391].

Because the organism is carried in 20% of healthy persons, the best test for disease is finding the toxin in the feces using the *C. difficile* toxin assay. Even then, the toxin assay is positive in only 70-80% of those with diarrhea due to *C. difficile*—70% after 1 specimen, 80% after 3 specimens. A newer enzyme immunoassay (EIA) is widely available now with similar sensitivity and specificity as the toxin assay. It is also much easier and quicker (2-4 hr vs. 1-2 days).

This disease should be considered anytime diarrhea occurs more than 6 days after initiation of antibiotics. Also suspect *C. difficile* infection in patients on antibiotics in whom unexplained leukocytosis (WBC > 15,000) develops.

Diagnosis of *C. difficile*: First do a fecal leukocyte (very sensitive). If fecal leukocyte positive, do an EIA (best) or toxin assay (good, just a long wait).

Treatment of *C. difficile*: stop the antibiotics and give metronidazole for 10 days. Previously oral vancomycin was the treatment of choice, but epidemics of vancomycin-resistant *Enterococcus faecium* have occurred because of this treatment! Additionally, metronidazole is as effective as vancomycin yet much less expensive. Relapse rate on either drug is about 10-20%. Because relapse is usually due to the spores becoming active, the proper treatment of a relapse is to just repeat the SAME treatment for the same duration. With multiple relapses, consider switching to vancomycin and consider tapering regimens of vancomycin after normal treatment to qd, then qod or q3d for a month. Bacitracin, rifampin, and cholestyramine are used as adjunctive therapy in complicated cases. Note that cholestyramine binds vancomycin and renders it ineffective.

Parasites

Amebic diarrhea may be acute or chronic. The stool may be watery or bloody and may or may not have fecal leukocytes. Occasionally this causes a fulminant colitis so rule this out before you put the patient on steroids for presumed IBD!! Most common extraintestinal manifestation is amebic liver abscess (immigrant or patient who has been out of the country with RUQ pain, fever, leukocytosis, increased LFTs, normal or slightly high bilirubin; only 1/3 have concurrent diarrhea).

Best screening is 3 stool specimens in preservative or in a dry container. Water and urine are dilute and destroy the ameba. Serology: counterimmune diffusion assay, agar gel diffusion assays, and ELISA. If serology is positive and the patient has a liver abscess, new colitis, or suspected ameboma, then the patient is treated for active amebic disease. This is proper because serologic findings usually revert to negative within 6 to 12 months. Indirect hemagglutination tests stay positive up to 10 years and interpretation is fuzzier (use the other tests if possible).

notes

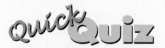

1) Which diarrheal organism is Guillain Barré most commonly linked to?

2) HUS associated with *E. coli* O157:H7 presents with what triad of symptoms?

3) Recurrence of *C. difficile* diarrhea warrants treatment with which agent?

4) What is the best way to diagnose giardial infection?

5) In an AIDS patient with fever and diarrhea, what organisms are on your differential list?

6) In an AIDS patient without fever and diarrhea, what are organisms on your differential?

7) Describe the diarrhea commonly seen with IBD involving the colon?

8) What are the symptoms of a secreting carcinoid?

9) Which type of carcinoid is most likely associated with hypotension?

10) How do you diagnose carcinoid?

Treatment is to aspirate and give metronidazole.

Giardiasis presents variably from asymptomatic carrier to self-limited acute diarrhea to acute progressive to chronic intermittent to chronic diarrhea. Symptoms begin 3-20 days after exposure. The diarrhea is associated with bloating, abdominal cramps, and a distinctive-smelling (whew!) flatus and frothy stool. Weight loss is frequent. It is best diagnosed with an enzyme-linked immunosorbent assay for Giardia antigen. This is both sensitive and specific (92% and 98%) and it becomes negative after successful therapy (i.e., this is an antigen test, not an antibody test). The classic series of 3 stool specimens is only 60-80% sensitive. The string test and biopsies are no longer required. Treat with quinacrine hydrochloride or metronidazole. Note: No eosinophilia, no stool WBCs or blood.

Cryptosporidiosis is a fairly common cause of sporadic gastroenteritis in immunocompetent persons and a very common cause of gastroenteritis in AIDS patients. Watery diarrhea with crampy epigastric pain are the predominant symptoms. No stool WBCs or blood. In the immunocompetent, it is usually self-limited—although it may take months. Not treated unless severe, then give paromomycin.

Chronic Diarrhea

Overview

II. Chronic secretory diarrhea has a high volume (> 1 L/day despite fasting), few (if any) fecal WBCs, and fecal 2[$Na^+ + K^+$] is approximately equal to the serum osmolality. Etiology: secretory tumors (e.g., villous adenomas), (low) bile acid-related diarrhea, and steatorrhea.

Special Note: Laxative abuse leads to an osmotic diarrhea with an osmotic gap > 50.

AIDS (know!): 60% of patients have diarrhea and weight loss. If the AIDS patient has diarrhea and weight loss without fever, suspect *Cryptosporidia* (usual cause), *E. histolytica*, *Giardia*, *Isospora*, *Strongyloides*, and AIDS enteropathy. Note that all these organisms are noninvasive. With fever, think of *Mycobacterium*, *Campylobacter*, *Salmonella*, *Cryptococcus*, *Histoplasma*, and CMV.

Volume is a big clue in AIDS-associated diarrhea. More than 1L/day suggests a small bowel cause.

A CD4 count < 200, especially if accompanied by weight loss, points to an infectious etiology rather than AIDS enteropathy.

IBD (know!): Chronic inflammatory disease of the colon (UC and Crohn colitis) causes a low volume diarrhea (or loose stools) with many WBCs. There is histologic damage. Chronic bloody diarrhea suggests UC. Chronic diarrhea associated with chronic RLQ abdominal cramping and especially palpation of thickened bowel in the RLQ suggest CD. Note that fecal WBCs and blood are found both in invasive diarrhea and UC.

Diabetic diarrhea may be caused by:
• Use of dietetic foods rich in sorbitol (erroneously labeled "sugarless").
• Visceral autonomic neuropathy (especially suspect this in the incontinent diabetic patient).
• Less common are various causes of malabsorption: sprue (present in 5% of diabetics), pancreatic insufficiency, and bacterial overgrowth (treat with metronidazole or amoxicillin-clavulanate).

Carbohydrate intolerance (lactose) or malabsorption (sorbitol, fructose) should be considered in all patients with chronic diarrhea.

Carcinoid is a less common cause of chronic diarrhea. Carcinoid is the most common intestinal neoplasm—by a factor of 10!! Most carcinoids are of the asymptomatic, nonsecreting type. Most nonsecreting carcinoids are found in the appendix. About 75% of the secreting, symptomatic carcinoids are in the ileum. Gastric carcinoids are related to hypergastrinemic states (this aspect discussed on pg 1-8).

The symptomatic carcinoids secrete various vasoactive mediators including 5-hydroxytryptophan, 5-hydroxytryptamine, and histamine which cause paroxysmal flushing; crampy, explosive diarrhea; and sometimes tachycardia and hypotension. The flushing is often bright red with well-defined borders and can be on the whole body—including hands and soles. The bronchial carcinoids (rare) cause more dramatic symptoms than the intestinal secreting type because the bronchial ones dump the vasoactive mediators directly into the arterial circulation. Because tryptophan, a precursor of niacin, is used up in carcinoid syndrome, niacin deficiency may occur.

Diagnosis: check 24 hour urine for 5-hydroxyindoleacetic acid (5-HIAA)—a breakdown product of 5-hydroxytryptamine.

notes

Normal is < 10 mg/24 hr; with carcinoid, patient has > 25 mg/24 hr.

Visceral autonomic neuropathy is characterized by:
- delayed gastric emptying (i.e., gastroparesis)
- postural decrease in blood pressure
- anhidrosis (inability to tolerate heat, lack of functioning sweat glands)
- fecal incontinence
- impotence (men)
- urinary overflow incontinence

Other causes of chronic diarrhea include previous surgery, steatorrhea (see next section), endocrine causes (hyper-& hypothyroidism, adrenal insufficiency), colon cancer, radiation-induced disease, and ischemic bowel disease.

Diagnosis of Chronic Diarrhea

Note that in the diagnosis of chronic diarrhea, as soon as the diagnosis is made, the testing is stopped:

Stage I: Stool O&P & fecal leukocytes x 3. Stool pH. *C. difficile* toxin assay. Weight of stool/24 hours. 3 day fecal fat (or if Sudan stain is positive, do the fecal fat). Also chem 20, thyroid profile, and gastrin level. Lactose free diet if lactase deficiency is at all suggested by history.

Stage II: Immunoabsorbent assay for giardiasis. If steatorrhea is confirmed, KUB for pancreatic calcification (discussed in detail in next section). If diabetic with suggestive history: either do a 14C-glycocholate breath test for bacterial overgrowth or (more often) just treat empirically. If > 1000 cc/d of stool, check vasoactive intestinal polypeptide. Also may do sigmoidoscopy and high quality UGI.

Laxative abuse is checked for by:
- specific urine tests for bisacodyl, anthraquinones, and phenolphthalein;
- stool osmotic gap > 100 (Mg);
- stool measurement of phosphate and sulfate.
- If the stool osmolality is low, the patient could be adding water or urine to the stool.

Stage III: EGD and colonoscopy.

If the patient has no determinable cause for the chronic diarrhea and does have abdominal pain, the diagnosis is probably irritable bowel syndrome (see pg 1-18). There are a significant number of patients who have no discernible cause of the diarrhea and have no abdominal pain. These patients have idiopathic chronic diarrhea. Often a hospital stay is required after phase III to redo and better control the previous tests.

MALABSORPTION

Overview

Malabsorption may be short-lived but patients often present with a chronic diarrhea. Malabsorption can be caused by **I**) decreased small bowel mucosal transport and by **II**) decreased digestion. As discussed more fully later, these are screened for with routine chemistries, looking for: LOW albumin, Ca^{++}, cholesterol, and/or carotene. We will now discuss the causes.

...Due to Decreased Mucosal Transport

I) Decreased mucosal transport: may be caused by celiac sprue, tropical sprue, hypogammaglobulinemic sprue, Whipple disease, intestinal lymphoma, eosinophilic gastroenteritis, bacterial overgrowth, and other small bowel disease. These are discussed below.

Celiac sprue (nontropical sprue; gluten-sensitive enteropathy)—malabsorption due to small bowel villous atrophy probably caused by an immune-mediated gluten sensitivity. It is prevalent in Ireland, it can cause growth retardation, and it is associated with HLA-B8. It may go into remission during adolescence, then recur. Patients may get dermatitis herpetiformis. The most common presentation (2000-2001) of celiac sprue patients is iron deficiency anemia (iron is absorbed mostly in the duodenum). Primary intestinal lymphoma is a rare late complication of celiac sprue.

Diagnosis of celiac sprue:
1) Evidence of malabsorption,
2) abnormal small bowel biopsy, and
3) a positive response to a gluten-free diet (clinical, chemical, and histological).

There are various antibody tests (IgA antiendomysial Ab [best], and IgG/IgA antigliadin Ab) which are specific but not sensitive enough for screening at-risk populations. These antibody tests may be useful for determining latent celiac sprue or as a measure of compliance with the gluten-free diet.

Note that these small bowel biopsy results are fairly nonspecific as similar villous atrophy is seen with hypogammaglobulinemia ("hypogammaglobulinemic sprue") and even acute gastroenteritis!

Treat with gluten free diet (GFD) +/- initial corticosteroids. 80% respond to a GFD although it may take awhile in some. For those patients NOT responding to a GFD, consider:
- noncompliance   • pancreatic insufficiency
- intestinal lymphoma   • collagenous sprue (see next)
- microscopic colitis.
- lactose intolerance 2° lactase deficiency (damaged mucosa)

Collagenous sprue is a possible variant of celiac sprue in which the small bowel biopsy shows flattened mucosa with large masses of subepithelial eosinophilic hyaline material in the lamina propria. About 30% of those with celiac sprue have some collagen deposition and 8% have dense deposition. More collagen deposition probably indicates worse prognosis.

Tropical sprue is a malabsorption with partial villous atrophy that is probably of an infectious etiology. It is endemic in areas of the Caribbean, S. Africa, Venezuela, India and S.E. Asia (i.e., the equatorial areas). Treatment: tetracycline or TMP/SMX for 3-6 months. Folic acid replacement has also been used either alone or as adjunctive treatment.

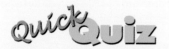

Quick Quiz

1) What are the three stages used in the workup of chronic diarrhea?

2) What is the most common clinical presentation for a patient with celiac sprue?

3) What are the findings for celiac sprue vs. tropical sprue? What are the treatments for each?

4) How may Whipple disease manifest when it relapses?

5) What must be ruled out in a patient older than 55 with pancreatic insufficiency?

6) Steatorrhea is the best indicator of _____?

7) What is the best test for steatorrhea?

8) Steatorrhea occurring as greater than 50 grams of fecal fat/day is almost always due to what?

9) Malabsorption may be due to problems with digestion or transport. Explain the properties of xylose that make it important in the diagnosis of malabsorption.

10) What is the significance of a normal D-xylose absorption test in a patient with steatorrhea? Low D-xylose?

Whipple disease—is probably caused by a gram-positive actinomycete recently found in the intestinal mucosa of patients with Whipple disease. It has been named *Tropheryma whippelii*. Infection causes weight loss, arthralgias, abdominal pain, diarrhea, and severe malabsorption—often with marked hypoalbuminemia. Some of these symptoms are caused by lymphatic obstruction. Small bowel biopsy shows specific foamy macrophages and positive for PAS-staining bacterial remnants. Treat with one year of antibiotics, especially TMP/SMX and tetracycline (often use two antibiotics)—also PCN or metronidazole may be included. Know that relapse often manifests with CNS symptoms.

DDx: These symptoms also may be caused by lymphatic blockage from primary intestinal (or other) lymphoma.

Eosinophilic gastroenteritis can mimic intestinal lymphoma and regional enteritis. Patients have N/V/diarrhea, abdominal pain, and weight loss, albumin wasting. They often have a peripheral eosinophilia and, even though it is thought to be due to an allergy to certain foods—which would be mediated by IgE—only 20% have specific food allergies with an increased IgE. Treat with corticosteroids and avoidance of the causative foods. Strongyloides can also cause a peripheral eosinophilia (Giardia does not) so be sure to rule this out before you start the steroids!

Short bowel syndrome occurs after massive resection of the small bowel usually due to
1) severe ischemic injury or
2) multiple surgeries for Crohn disease and jejunoileal bypass for morbid obesity.

Short bowel syndrome is likely when there is less than (roughly) 2 feet of small bowel—especially when the proximal jejunum and/or distal ileum are involved. Susceptible to calcium oxalate kidney stones and gastric acid hypersecretion. Treated with a low fat diet and vitamin supplements. TPN may be needed after large resection while waiting hopefully for bowel adaptation.

...Due to Decreased Digestion

II) Decreased digestion. Two main causes:

1) Pancreatic insufficiency: as can be seen in chronic pancreatitis, pancreatic cancer, and cystic fibrosis. Pancreatic insufficiency is determined by the qualitative stool exam revealing undigested muscle fibers, neural fat, and split fat. The undigested muscle fibers indicates impaired digestion. Impaired digestion is further confirmed by a positive response to treatment with pancreatic enzymes. The xylose absorption test may also be done during the workup (discussed below) and is normal.

You must rule out pancreatic cancer if there is evidence of pancreatic insufficiency in patients > 55 years old.

2) Bile acid deficiency: a) Ileal resection or disease that decreases bile acid uptake. b) Severe liver disease which decreases production of bile acids. c) Zollinger-Ellison syndrome in which the patient has increased acidity in the small bowel which precipitates the bile acids. d) Bacterial overgrowth resulting in the breakdown of bile acids making them useless for fat digestion. Discussed below.

Steatorrhea is the best indicator of any type of malabsorption because it usually is the most prominent problem. Sudan stain of the stool (for fat) is the best screening test. Serum carotene levels are a less specific indicator for malabsorption (see next). The 3-day, quantitative fecal fat measurement is the "gold standard" for determining steatorrhea. Because diarrhea itself can cause up to 14 g/d fecal fat, steatorrhea is defined as > 14 gm/d of fecal fat. Steatorrhea from pancreatic insufficiency causes the most fecal fat (can be > 50 gm/d!); any patient having > 40 gm/d of fecal fat almost certainly has pancreatic insufficiency.

Cause: Digestion vs. Transport

Diagnosing etiology of the malabsorption: First you should determine whether it is a small bowel mucosal problem or pancreatic insufficiency (transport vs. digestion). This is determined using the xylose absorption test. Xylose requires normal transmucosal transport but it does not require digestion by pancreatic enzymes to be absorbed.

Know!: A normal xylose absorption test result (> 4.5 gm of a 25 gm oral dose should be excreted in the urine over 5 hr or patient has a > 20 mg/dl serum level) in a patient with steatorrhea excludes diffuse small bowel disease (celiac sprue, short bowel syndrome, etc.) and makes pancreatic insufficiency more likely. These patients are often empirically treated with pancreatic enzymes. Resolution of the symptoms is both therapeutic and confirms the diagnosis. Note: normal

notes

urinary xylose after a 25 gm oral load is 6.0 +/- 1.5 gm over 5hr.

On the other hand, a low result (< 5 gm) can be caused not only by small bowel disease but also by many other conditions including poor gastric emptying, bacterial overgrowth, ascites, renal insufficiency, and old age! But, if the patient definitely has steatorrhea, the likelihood is that the diagnosis is small bowel disease since most of the other causes of an abnormal D-xylose test do not cause steatorrhea. So, D-xylose low?...do a small bowel biopsy!

The absorption of carotene, vitamin K, vitamin D, folate, and iron are also, like xylose, independent of pancreatic enzyme digestion. So, chronic non-bloody diarrhea with low serum carotene, hypocalcemia, hypoprothrombinemia, and/or Fe deficiency anemia suggests a small bowel malabsorption problem rather than pancreatic disorder—this is true only if the patient has a normal dietary intake and only after prolonged disease. Conversely, chronic diarrhea and normal levels of the above indicates pancreatic insufficiency. An alcoholic who has an elevated prothrombin time easily corrected by vitamin K more likely has malabsorption as the cause of the high PT, not liver disease!

Combined Causes

The above causes of malabsorption can be combined as in bacterial overgrowth which results in bile acid deconjugation and variable patchy destruction of intestinal villi. It occurs in a variety of conditions:
- Structural abnormalities—(diverticula, fistulae, strictures, post ileocecal resection),
- Motility disorders—peristalsis is a major mechanism for clearing the small intestine of bacteria (may be defective in diabetes and scleroderma).
- Achlorhydria—acid in the stomach kills bacteria before it enters the small bowel.
- Immune disorders—immunoglobulins secreted in small bowel may decrease bacterial growth.

There is associated moderate steatorrhea. Diagnosis: Bacterial overgrowth can be diagnosed with the C^{14}-glycocholate breath test and the lactulose breath test. Contrary to other causes of malabsorption, these patients often have an increased RBC folate level. These tests are usually available only at large medical centers. Bacterial overgrowth is often treated empirically.

IRRITABLE BOWEL SYNDROME

A large part of a Gastroenterologist's practice consists of functional complaints. About 15% of the population has signs/symptoms of irritable bowel syndrome (IBS) and by far the majority are women. IBS has characteristic symptoms of frequent, small stools with mucus and abdominal pain relieved by defecation. These symptoms may be either continuous or recurring. There are no nocturnal symptoms nor organic symptoms. Patients generally have an increased bowel motor response to emotional and physical stimuli but these motor patterns are not specific to IBS. IBS patients are more likely to have been abused in childhood.

The diagnosis of IBS is derived by a combination of excluding other diseases and looking for characteristic symptoms. Rule out sorbitol use, lactose intolerance, and do a sigmoidoscopy (not colonoscopy) to help exclude IBD. The characteristic symptom pattern of the abdominal pain and changed bowel habits has been formalized into the International Classification for Irritable Bowel Syndrome—usually called the Rome criteria. These are (know):

At least 3 months of continuous or recurrent:
1) Abdominal pain relieved by defecation or accompanied by a change in frequency or consistence of stool
   and
2) Disturbed defecation at least 25% of the time consisting of 2 or more:
   - Altered frequency   • Altered consistency
   - Passage of mucus   • Altered stool passage
   - Abdominal distention
     and
3) No constitutional signs or symptoms such as fever, weight loss, anorexia, and anemia.

The drug of choice for treatment of IBS depends on the clinical presentation. Initially, education and reassurance along with dietary modification and fiber supplementation are indicated. That reassurance is paramount is shown by the very impressive 60-70% (!) response to placebo these patients have—although only 30% have *adequate* relief with placebo. If this treatment fails then, depending on signs and symptoms, the following are used: antispasmodic (anticholinergic) agents, antidiarrheals, tricyclic antidepressants, anxiolytics, and prokinetics.

If the symptoms are associated with eating or defecation, a motility drug is used. If there are psychological factors, give a psychoactive drug. For example, if the patient has signs or symptoms of depression or a neurosis, a tricyclic is often given. If the patient has fecal urgency and soiling, loperamide is given (it decreases motility and increases sphincter tone). If symptoms follow eating, an anticholinergic like dicyclomine is given.

INTESTINAL CANCER
OVERVIEW

Colon cancer risk factors: Age > 50; history of adenomatous polyps; history of breast, ovarian, or endometrial cancer; 1st degree relatives with colon cancer or adenomatous polyps; the familial polyposis (FP) syndromes (see next); ulcerative colitis; Crohn's colitis; and daily meat ingestion.

Decreased risk for both men and women: 4+ aspirin 325 mg tabs per week for 20+ years. Little if any benefit at less than 20 years; you should not be asked about this because studies with < 20 years of use have conflicting results.

notes

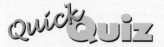

1) How do you diagnose bacterial overgrowth as a cause of diarrhea?

2) A 23 year old patient has had 8 weeks of abdominal pain and distention relieved by frequent mucousy bowel movements (75%). Is this irritable bowel?

3) Endocarditis due to _____ or _____ (organisms) warrant a colonoscopy to search for colon carcinoma.

4) True or False: Hyperplastic polyps have malignant potential.

5) What size and histology findings of colon adenomas are considered "advanced features" with increased malignant potential?

6) Which 2 familial polyposis syndromes have the highest risk of carcinoma? Which has NO risk of carcinoma?

7) Why does Peutz-Jeghers syndrome have a risk of cancer even though it consists of hamartomas?

8) Colon cancer screening: When is a flex-sig indicated for a patient > 50 years? When is a colonoscopy?

The diagnostic flags:
- anorexia
- weight loss
- anemia
- fever
- heme+ stools
- nocturnal stools
- onset of symptoms after age 45

Also remember endocarditis caused by either *Strep bovis* and *Clostridium septicus* are often associated with colon cancer, so a thorough GI check is indicated in these patients.

Most GI cancers arise from adenomas. Most, but not all, adenomatous polyps occur in the rectosigmoid area. Adenomas with "advanced" features are defined as:

1) > 1 cm (see Table 1-4).
2) histology is <u>villous</u> or tubulo<u>villous</u>. (Note: just tubular is benign)

Advanced means likely to cause cancer. Progression to cancer from an early adenoma takes 5-10 years. Diet plays a role in GI cancer—possible dietary factors include high animal fats, low fiber, and low calcium in the diet.

Again, LARGE and VILLOUS polyps cause CANCER.

Hyperplastic polyps have no malignant potential and contain no features of dysplasia. This makes sense because hyperplasia by definition is increased growth of normal tissue.

Table 1-4: Malignant potential vs size

	< 1 cm	1-2 cm	> 2 cm
TUBULAR	1%	10%	34%
MIXED (TV)	4%	9%	45%
VILLOUS	10%	10%	54%

FAMILIAL POLYPOSIS SYNDROMES

Colon Cancer Families: Polyposis vs. Nonpolyposis syndromes.

The <u>Familial (or hereditary) Polyposis Syndromes</u> are all autosomal dominant (AD) [pg 132, #394-396]. In order of decreasing cancer potential:

1) Familial colonic polyposis—hundreds of adenomas in the colon—100% risk of cancer if not treated—these patients require a proctocolectomy at age 20!

2) Gardner syndrome—multiple colonic and occasional duodenal adenomas. Risk of cancer is also 100%. These patients often have bone lesions (osteomas) and soft tissue tumors. Treatment is the same as familial colonic polyposis. Question: Patient has multiple osteomas found incidentally on an x-ray. What do you do? Colonoscopy!

3) Peutz-Jeghers syndrome—multiple hamartomatous polyps throughout the small bowel and occasionally in the colorectum and stomach plus melanotic pigmentation (freckles) on the lips and buccal mucosa. Even though these polyps are hamartomas, there is still some risk of cancer because there are still occasional adenomas which can become carcinomas. The most common presentation is with abdominal pain due to intussusception or bowel obstruction by a large polyp.

4) Juvenile polyposis also consists of hamartomas. This is the only one of these syndromes with no malignant potential. No follow-up needed.

HEREDITARY <u>NON</u>-POLYPOSIS COLON CANCER

However, affected persons in most colon cancer families do not have familial polyposis—rather the cancer arises from normal-appearing epithelium. Hereditary nonpolyposis colon cancer (HNPCC or Lynch syndrome) can be defined as "the occurrence of colon cancer in at least three 1st degree relatives over at least two generations and with at least one person diagnosed under the age of 50." This rather loose diagnostic criteria places Lynch syndrome on as many as 1 in 200 people!! Women in families with HNPCC often have greatly increased incidence of <u>ovarian</u> and endometrial cancer.

SCREENING

Review

Current screening recommendations for low risk patients are to do yearly rectal exams and fecal occult blood testing (FOBT), and flex-sig every 3-5 years after age 50.

The recommendations stating the use of a flex-sig are probably going to change soon. New data show that flex-sig and FOBT miss 25% of colonic polyps. Absence of polyps in the distal colon is no guarantee of absence elsewhere in the colon. Also finding hyperplastic polyps distally is no guarantee that there are no adenomatous polyps proximally. Only a colonoscopy can do an adequate survey of the colon.

notes

If flexible sigmoidoscopy reveals a polyp, biopsy it! A full colonoscopy is then indicated if the polyp has "advanced" features (discussed earlier: 1) size > 1.0 cm or 2) histology showing villous or tubulovillous architecture). Repeat colonoscopy every 3 years thereafter if benign.

Plain tubular and hyperplastic are not advanced features; they are benign.

Increased risk patients: onset of surveillance (colonoscopy) should be at age 50 years or 10 years before age at which index case is diagnosed—whichever is first.

For example: Start at age 40 if a first degree relative was diagnosed with an adenoma or colon cancer at age 50, etc.

Colonoscopy is the screening procedure of choice if 1 or more 1st degree relatives have had colon cancer or an adenomatous polyp or if an adenomatous polyp has ever been found in the patient. Time between surveillance colonoscopy is dependent on the cancer potential of the polyp: 1-2 years after a less benign polyp but still every 3-5 years for more benign polyps.

Sigmoid colon cancer can perforate the bowel wall and simulate diverticulitis. So survey for colon cancer after diverticulitis in older patients.

FOBT

Fecal occult blood testing (FOBT). FOBT is positive in 1-15% of non-rehydrated samples. Of those, about 10% have GI neoplasms—and many of these neoplasms are POLYPS. So if there is positive FOBT do a colonoscopy. A flex-sig + ACBE (air contrast BE) is also acceptable but less desirable.

Remember that the FOBT is negative in half of patients with GI cancer. This makes it a pretty poor screening test but it is used (annually to biennially) because it is quick and cheap. The ACP, in its position paper (Annals 1997; 126) does not recommend rehydration of samples as it increases sensitivity at the cost of decreasing specificity. Probability of cancer in positive rehydrated screens is 2-3% whereas it is 10-15% in positive non-rehydrated screens—leading to vastly more colonoscopies (I suspect many GI docs like rehydration!) .

CEA

Note that carcinoembryonic antigen (CEA) levels are only good in checking for recurrence of colon cancer—and only if levels were elevated before surgery and reduced after surgery. CEA may also be mildly elevated in patients who smoke or who have benign biliary disease, sclerosing cholangitis, or inflammatory bowel disease.

DUKES CLASSIFICATION

Duke's classification of colorectal cancer reflects how the depth of penetration and the amount of spread affects prognosis. Colon cancer illustrations: [pg 133, #397-398]

Duke stage A is cancer confined to the mucosa and submucosa—with treatment, 5 year survival is 95%.

Stage B is cancer extending to the muscularis (B1) or through the serosa (B2)—this decreases 5 year survival to 70% (B1) and 85% (B2).

Stage C is when the cancer extends to the regional lymph nodes—5 year survival is about 35-65%. C1 = 1-4 nodes; C2 = 5 or more nodes.

Stage D is with distant metastases—5 year survival is only 5%. Colon cancer virtually always metastasizes to the liver first (via portal circulation). If it involves the rectum, it can bypass the portal circulation and so the patient may have lung, bone and brain mets without liver mets.

TREATMENT for INTESTINAL CANCER

Treatment for intestinal cancer consists of surgery. Surgery for cure in Dukes A and B. Surgery with adjuvant chemotherapy in Dukes C increased survival to 60% compared to 40% with surgery alone. Surgery is only palliative in stage D.

The adjuvant chemotherapy consists of 5-FU + levamisole. Levamisole has no anti-cancer effect itself; it potentiates the effect of the 5-FU. There is no added benefit using 5-FU for Dukes stage A or B. Again: adjuvant chemo only for Dukes C.

Radiation therapy prior to surgery is helpful for rectal lesions only. Hepatic resection increases survival for solitary liver mets.

If you remove a polyp which has cancer, you must do a bowel resection if the cancer extends to either a blood vessel or to the cautery line.

Review: Adenocarcinoma = Crohn and Familial polyposis syndromes. Lymphoma = sprue.

DIVERTICULAR DISEASE and LOWER GI BLEED
OVERVIEW

Diverticular disease—4 types:
1) Asymptomatic diverticulosis (most common) [pg 131, #392-393],
2) Painful diverticulosis (contraction of hypertrophied colonic muscle),
3) Diverticular bleeding [pg 134, #401],
4) Diverticulitis.

Diverticular bleeding usually originates in the sigmoid colon and it usually stops spontaneously. Patients classically present with "painless maroon stool" but it can vary from black to red. Diverticular bleeding is the most common cause of colonic bleeding in the elderly; angiodysplasia is next on the list and often results in more severe bleeds. Treatment: Stabilize patient if needed, rule out UGI bleed with NG aspirate or endoscopy.

notes

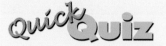

Note: UGI bleed is suggested by a BUN/Cr ratio > 30:1, which indicates blood is being digested.

Diagnose diverticular bleeding with endoscopy, technetium tagged RBC scan, or angiography works if bleeding is severe or continuous.

Diverticulitis is usually due to microperforations. Younger individuals tend to have more severe and more frequent episodes. Signs and symptoms:
1) LLQ pain 2) Fever 3) High WBC 4) LLQ tenderness—may be localized rebound tenderness.

Look for signs of a sigmoid mass on physical exam, U/S, or CT. CT scan determines if there is an abscess and is only indicated in more severe episodes. Avoid GI endoscopy on any patient with diverticulitis.

Treatment of diverticulitis should cover gram-negative and anaerobic organisms. Diverticulitis in a patient able to drink and without peritoneal signs may be treated with outpatient metronidazole + ciprofloxacin and close follow-up. Inpatient treatment for those with peritoneal signs may consist of:
1) dual drug therapy such as aminoglycoside + clindamycin, or
2) single drug therapy such as cefoxitin, ticarcillin-clavulanic acid, or imipenem-cilastatin.

Abscesses are usually drained percutaneously.

Perforation from sigmoid colon cancer can present similarly, so with patients > 50, follow up with a flex-sig/colonoscopy after the acute condition resolves.

Meckel diverticulum is the most frequent congenital GI anomaly. Although less than half of these diverticula have gastric mucosa, only these ulcerate and bleed. Meckel diverticula cause half of all GI bleeds in children. It can also cause obstruction and intussusception. They may be seen with the technetium scan ("Meckel's scan"). Technetium is taken up by gastric mucosa.

ANGIODYSPLASIA and LOWER GI BLEED

Angiodysplasia (= vascular ectasia, = AVM) is a common cause of lower GI bleeding in the elderly. Think of these as spider nevi of the GI tract. The bleeding may be occult to severe. Usual bleeding site is the right colon. Hereditary hemorrhagic telangiectasias (Osler-Rendu-Weber) is the hereditary condition in which there are multiple AVMs affecting all the organs including brain, lung, skin and mucous membranes, and GI tract—especially in the upper GI tract. Treatment is laser photocoagulation, electrocautery, or injection of a sclerosing agent.

BOWEL OBSTRUCTION

Obstruction: The most frequent cause of small intestine obstruction is post-operative adhesions. In decreasing order, the most common causes of colonic obstruction are: carcinoma… then diverticulitis…then volvulus. Know that the diagnosis of obstruction is made with a flat and upright abdominal film showing (typically) excessive amounts of free air in the small bowel with no air in the colon. The presence of air fluid levels is helpful when there are "J-loops" in which the air fluid levels are at different heights on either side of the same loop of bowel. This signifies a dynamic obstruction. If the fluid levels are the same height on either side of the loop, paralytic ileus is the more likely diagnosis. Usual treatment is IV fluids and ng suction. Further workup if the symptoms do not resolve in 1-2 days. Gastrografin enema can be helpful if the obstruction is thought to be of colonic origin.

INTESTINAL ISCHEMIA

Types

Intestinal Ischemia. 4 types: Colonic ischemia, chronic and acute mesenteric ischemia, and mesenteric venous thrombosis.

Colonic Ischemia

1) Colonic ischemia (CI; ischemic colitis). This is due to a non-occlusive ischemia—mostly involving some portions of the splenic flexure, descending colon, and/or sigmoid colon (i.e., inferior mesenteric circulation). Most often, no specific cause for the ischemia is found although it is a disease of the elderly and is occasionally associated with low flow conditions (CHF) and hypercoagulable states. As this condition is virtually never embolic, patients are not likely to have valvular heart disease or cardiac arrhythmia.

Symptoms of CI are usually a sudden LLQ pain with an urge to defecate followed by passage of red to maroon stool within 1 day.

Mildest injury is mucosal and submucosal hemorrhage and edema—which is completely reversible. More severe injury ranges from replacement of the mucosa and submucosa with

notes

Table 1-5: Angiography in GI disease
USE OF ANGIOGRAPHY IN GI DISEASE
Chronic and acute mesenteric ischemia
Severe lower GI bleed
Rarely used for UGI bleed - some duodenal ulcers
TIPS in variceal bleeding
Therapeutic uses: embolization, vasopressin

granulation tissue to transmural infarction and fulminant colitis.

Submucosal hemorrhage is seen on KUB or BE as "thumbprinting" [(pg 134, #400)]. This thumbprinting lasts only a few days. Angiography has little value. Diagnostic procedure of choice, if there are no signs of peritonitis, is colonoscopy. Also okay is sigmoidoscopy + gentle barium enema. The usual treatment is bowel rest, fluids, and antibiotics. With this treatment, 50% of patients have complete resolution, 30% heal with stricture, and 20% get a gangrenous gut. If no relief, surgical intervention is indicated.

Chronic Mesenteric Ischemia

2) Chronic mesenteric ischemia is also termed intestinal angina. These patients may have the classic triad:
• Abdominal pain after meals
• Abdominal bruit
• Weight loss (from tolerating only smaller meals)

An arteriogram is indicated if mesenteric ischemia is suspected. If this is positive, surgery or angioplasty is indicated. Symptoms are 1-3 hours of dull, gnawing abdominal pain beginning shortly after eating. The cause is atherosclerosis of the intestinal arteries with the symptoms being caused by gastric "steal" after eating. Patients often have signs of other PVD and often have a smoking history. Diagnosis is based on symptoms and angiography (or MRI angiography) with evidence of occlusion in the splanchnic (intestinal) arteries. Only treatment is surgical bypass. Angioplasty is being evaluated.

Acute Mesenteric Ischemia

3) Acute mesenteric ischemia results from acute loss of blood flow to part or all of the small intestine and/or ascending colon. Seen in older patients with a history of CHF, recent MI, cardiac arrhythmias, or hypotensive episodes. Patients often have symptoms of intestinal angina (above) for months before the event. As this condition is commonly embolic, patients are likely to have valvular heart disease or cardiac arrhythmia. These patients are acutely ill with vomiting, diarrhea, occult blood. If there is bowel perforation, chemistry may show acidosis, increased SGOT (ALT), and elevated amylase. The abdominal exam may be fairly benign leading to the erroneous diagnosis of acute gastroenteritis. Angiography is done unless there are signs of perforation (e.g., acido-

Table 1-6: Indications for Colonoscopy
COLONOSCOPY - INDICATIONS
Occult Bleeding
Fe deficiency anemia in a man
Gross lower GI bleeding except bright red blood in a younger person
Abnormal barium enema
Adenomatous polyp - initially and for all followups
History of colon cancer
1st degree relative of one with colon cancer
FCP, HNPCC/Lynch
IBD: suspicion, followup, surveillance
Strep bovis, Clostridium septicum
Ischemic colitis (sometimes)
Persistent diarrhea with negative blood tests and not meeting criteria for diagnosis of IBS

sis, high amylase)—in which case the patient goes directly to surgery for dead bowel resection and possible embolectomy.

Mesenteric Venous Thrombosis

4) Mesenteric venous thrombosis (MVT) is associated with
• hypercoagulable states such as deficiencies of antithrombin III, prothrombin 20210 (a gene variant), protein S, and protein C and factor V Leiden defect.

MVT is also linked to
• pancreatitis   • liver disease   • intraabdominal sepsis

MVT may be acute, subacute, or chronic. Like mesenteric infarction, the pain of MVT is often out of proportion to the abdominal exam. If the portal or splenic veins are involved in chronic MVT, there may be bleeding from gastroesophageal varices. CT is the diagnostic procedure of choice—with it > 90% of MVT can be diagnosed. Treat acute MVT with thrombolytics and long-term anticoagulants. Treatment of chronic MVT is focused on minimizing bleeding from varices with sclerotherapy, portosystemic shunts, etc.

CONSTIPATION

Causes of constipation are vast but usually result in abnormal colonic transit or abnormal anorectal function. Know that the large majority of cases are idiopathic. Lifestyle changes such as a change to low fiber diet, sudden prolonged inactivity, and high stress may result in constipation. Typically these

notes

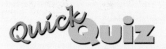
can be diagnosed from a careful history. Treatment is covered below.

Recent onset of constipation (no changes to diet, no new medications, etc.) suggests an obstructing lesion (neoplasm, stricture, foreign body). Pelvic floor dysfunction acts like outlet obstruction. This often responds to pelvic floor retraining (with biofeedback). Know that hysterectomy leads to refractory constipation in 5% of patients.

Neurologic causes affecting the parasympathetic innervation of the distal colon and rectum cause acquired megacolon. E.g., traumatic sacral nerve damage, multiple sclerosis (MS), Chagas disease, or aganglionic megacolon (Hirschsprung). Chagas disease is found in Central and S. America. It is caused by infection with *Trypanosoma cruzi* resulting in achalasia, cardiomyopathy, and acquired megacolon. Aganglionic megacolon (Hirschsprung) is usually diagnosed within the first 6 months of life but a milder variant may present in adult patients.

Drugs with anticholinergic properties are common causes of constipation. These include antipsychotics, antidepressants, first-generation antihistamines, and anticholinergic cold medications. Other causes include iron preparations, calcium supplements and calcium-channel blockers, and antacids containing aluminum or calcium.

Endocrine disorders such as diabetes mellitus and hypothyroidism often cause mild constipation. Myxedema may result in acquired megacolon. The altered progesterone and estrogen levels are the probable cause of constipation in pregnancy.

Collagen vascular diseases: especially progressive systemic sclerosis.

Diagnosis in intractable constipation: In general sigmoidoscopy and/or BE (not colonoscopy—overkill) is the first step.

Treatment consists of correcting any reversible cause. If idiopathic or irreversible, treatment is increasing dietary fiber to 25-30 gm/day. Increase exercise. Short-term use of an osmotic laxative and/or stool softener is okay. Avoid stimulant laxatives. Surgical treatment is indicated only for Hirschsprung disease.

PANCREAS

ACUTE PANCREATITIS

Overview

Acute pancreatitis is usually caused by either alcohol abuse or gallstones. In the U.S., the primary cause of acute pancreatitis is thought to be alcohol, followed by gallstones. In Europe, the reverse appears to be true. These are not firm conclusions; results from studies are influenced by where they are done. For example, if the study is done in a VA hospital, the primary cause will probably be alcohol abuse whereas, if it is done in a community hospital, gallstones are more likely to cause the majority of cases.

Other causes of acute pancreatitis are acidosis (as in DKA), hypertriglyceridemia, hypercalcemia, trauma, and other problems that result in obstruction of the ampulla of Vater, such as pancreatic cancer [pg 127, #381]. Acute pancreatitis follows ERCP in 2-8%. Quite a few drugs can cause acute pancreatitis:
- diuretics: furosemide and the thiazides
- estrogen
- azathioprine
- antibiotics: tetracycline and the sulfonamides
- anti-HIV drugs such as: pentamidine, ddI, and ddC.
- also implicated are oral hypoglycemics, 6-mercaptopurine, L-asparaginase, and valproic acid

Many "idiopathic" cases are due to biliary microlithiasis or cystic fibrosis.

With acute pancreatitis, amylase and lipase are usually elevated. The serum amylase level is almost always elevated early on (> 3xN is almost always due to pancreatitis) but decreases within 2-3 days after disease onset. The lipase level increases later and stays elevated longer than the amylase—7-14 days. Hypertriglyceridemia may cause spuriously normal amylase and levels! Very elevated serum or urine amylase levels, >900 U/L and > 6000 U/L respectively, are very specific indicators of acute pancreatitis (97%) but they have low sensitivity (50-70%).

Again: High triglyceride level in the setting of acute pancreatitis may cause a spuriously normal amylase level! Triglyceride levels > 1000 mg/dL are associated with an increased risk of acute pancreatitis.

Mortality rate for acute pancreatitis = 10%! The severity of acute pancreatitis is thought to be a direct result of the degree of pancreatic necrosis and whether it is infected (mortality = 30%) or not (mortality = 10%). Pancreatic necrosis is best diagnosed by dynamic CT scan. This is considered severe if ≥ 30% of the pancreas is necrotic. Severe pancreatic necrosis causes multiple organ failure reflected by:
- Heart: systolic BP < 90 mmHg; tachycardia > 130 bpm,
- Lungs: PO_2 < 60 mmHg,

- Renal: progressive azotemia *or* oliguria<50 mL/hr,
- CNS = altered sensorium,
- Metabolic = low calcium (< 8 mg/dL) and albumin. <3.2 g/dL

Two factors indicate that a patient is more likely to have severe pancreatitis:
1) overweight with a BMI > 25 (especially if obese with BMI of > 29), and
2) hemoconcentration with Hct > 50%.

Risk Factors

These signs of organ failure are used in the APACHE II system in which severe pancreatitis is indicated by a score of > 8-12. The APACHE II score is more sensitive and specific than the Ranson/Imrie criteria but requires a computer to figure and therefore is not embraced by many. It *is* used in ICUs. Note that the presence of any two of the above findings of severe necrosis (except altered sensorium) is associated with a 20-30% mortality.

The Ranson/Imrie criteria: Increased severity if 3 or more of the following risk factors are found on admission or in first 48 hours (these don't require a computer):

Risk factors on admission:
- increased age
- high WBC
- hyperglycemia
- first attack
- abdominal mass
- discolored peritoneal fluid
- hypotension
- abnormal lung findings

Infected pancreatic necrosis is more likely to develop (30%!!) if there are 3 or more Ranson's criteria.

Risk factors during the first 48 hours:
- hypotension and persistent tachycardia,
- hypovolemia and need for > 4L fluid replacement,
- hematocrit dropping > 10% with hydration,
- hypocalcemia (<8 mg/dL),
- hypoxia +/- ARDS,
- hypoalbuminemia (<3.2)
- BUN incr > 5 mg/dL.

Here, dehydration is defined as > 10% fall in Hct with hydration. Hypocalcemia is not treated in this setting—it is from sequestration, not a decrease in total body stores.

Note: Cullen sign and Turner sign, when seen (unusual), indicate a severe necrotizing pancreatitis. Cullen sign, a faint blue discoloration around the umbilicus, may occur as the result of hemoperitoneum, while Turner's sign, a bluish-reddish-purple or greenish-brown discoloration of the flanks, results from tissue catabolism of hemoglobin.

New indicators predicting severity in pancreatitis are being tested. Urinary assay of trypsinogen activation peptide (TAP) 24 hours after onset of symptoms provides an accurate severity prediction. C-reactive protein is not as good as TAP and provided no benefit when used with TAP. Serum granulocyte elastase is being evaluated.

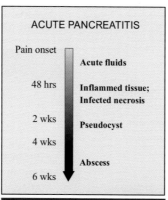

ACUTE PANCREATITIS

Pain onset

48 hrs — Acute fluids

Inflamed tissue; Infected necrosis

2 wks — Pseudocyst

4 wks

Abscess

6 wks

Figure 1-3: Timeline of Complications

In working up the cause of acute pancreatitis, the first test is gallbladder ultrasound.

Fluid/masses in acute pancreatitis:

- Acute fluid collections with high amylase levels appear in up to 50% of patients within 48 hours of pain onset. They usually resolve spontaneously. A sympathetic transudative left pleural effusion frequently occurs. Rarely, a fistula forms into the pleural space causing an effusion high in amylase. (See Figure 1-3)
- Inflamed, edematous pancreatic tissue also occurs early on and it may simulate a mass. It should be aspirated to check for infection. It usually resolves spontaneously.
- Infected pancreatic necrosis requires surgery. It occurs within 2 weeks of the episode. It can be diagnosed by CT-guided aspiration of necrotic pancreas with bacterial smear and culture.
- A pancreatic pseudocyst develops in 10-15% of patients with acute pancreatitis. It requires 1-4 weeks to develop after the acute attack. Basically it is a collection of pancreatic fluid which, if small enough, resolves spontaneously. A size > 5 cm suggests it may not resolve. If the pseudocyst persists > 3-6 month, it will probably require surgical drainage [(pg 143, #427)]. Pseudocysts must be removed as they are associated with serious complications—especially fistula, pseudoaneurysms, rupture, and hemorrhage. Rupture without hemorrhage has a 15% mortality while rupture with hemorrhage has a 60% mortality!
- A pancreatic abscess develops over a longer period than infected pancreatic necrosis—often 4-6 weeks after onset of acute pancreatitis. It may be seen as a "soap bubble sign" on upright abdominal x-ray. Diagnosis is by gram stain of a CT-directed percutaneous aspiration—which is 90% accurate. This allows early diagnosis and treatment (immediate surgical debridement and drainage) and improved survival.

Treatment of Acute Pancreatitis

Treatment: About 90% resolve spontaneously within a few days with supportive care. Patients must be made NPO, but NG suction is generally not required. IV fluids and colloids as needed.

Systemic antibiotics are given if there is severe pancreatitis with any organ failure or ≥ 30% pancreatic necrosis. Use antibiotics excreted in the pancreas, e.g., imipenem or cefuroxime.

Pearls of Acute Pancreatitis

Acute pancreatitis pearls.
1) If the amylase is still elevated after 10 days, think of something else going on such as a (leaking?) pseudocyst or disrupted main pancreatic duct.

notes

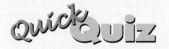

2) Recurrent acute pancreatitis with no evidence of gallstones or alcohol abuse may be due to microlithiasis and an elective cholecystectomy should be considered.

3) Gastric varices in the absence of esophageal varices occur only in splenic vein thrombosis which is a complication of both severe acute pancreatitis and chronic pancreatitis.

4) ERCP is not done acutely unless a patient has cholangitis and sepsis. ERCP after the acute period is used to exclude or treat any suspected common duct stones (e.g., the bilirubin is > 2.5 or the ultrasound shows a dilated common duct). Cholecystectomy should be done ASAP after gallstone pancreatitis.

Question: What conditions can cause abdominal pain with an elevated amylase? Answer: Acute pancreatitis, acute cholecystitis, intestinal infarction, diabetic ketoacidosis, perforated ulcer, salpingitis, and ectopic pregnancy! Other causes of hyperamylasemia are increased salivary amylase and macroamylasemia (a benign condition due to a low urinary excretion of amylase).

CHRONIC PANCREATITIS

Overview

Chronic pancreatitis is, in developed countries, usually (60-70%) a result of chronic alcohol ingestion—usually for > 10 years. Next in frequency is idiopathic (30%). Other causes include cystic fibrosis, pancreas divisum, tumor, and hyperparathyroidism. There is an asymptomatic initial phase followed by recurrent bouts of abdominal pain. Late in the disease, when > 80-90% of the endocrine and exocrine function is lost, the patients develop steatorrhea and diabetes. The fecal fat in these late stage patients is higher than with other disorders—it may be > 100 gm/day. Greater than 40 gm/day is highly suggestive of chronic pancreatitis. One third of patients with chronic pancreatitis develop diabetes (see below).

Chronic pancreatitis also increases the risk of pancreatic cancer [pg 143, #428-429].

Diagnosis

The classic diagnostic triad for chronic pancreatitis is:
• Pancreatic calcification
• Diabetes
• Steatorrhea

Diagnosis can be difficult and evaluation should begin with simple, noninvasive tests which detect advanced forms of chronic pancreatis. First get a flat plate x-ray of the abdomen and a serum trypsin level—if the pancreas is calcified, or if the serum trypsin is abnormally low, the diagnosis of chronic pancreatitis is made! Second level tests, if needed, are abdominal U/S or CT, bentiromide testing (Chymex—no longer available in the U.S.), or the secretin stimulation testing (see below). If still negative, and the diagnosis is still suspected, then an ERCP is indicated (90% sensitive). The ERCP may show large duct disease _or_ small duct disease. With large duct disease, pancreatic duct has stenoses and dilations which, on ERCP with retrograde pancreatography, visualize as an irregular "chain of lakes."

Dilation of the common bile duct can be caused by chronic pancreatitis but also by pancreatic cancer: either can compress the downstream portion of the common bile duct as it passes through the head of the pancreas.

The secretin test is the most sensitive test for pancreatic function but it is complicated, so is usually performed only in major medical centers and only when there is still a high "index of suspicion" after a negative ERCP (this does vary—in some places with ready access, it is done before ERCP). In this test, IV infusion of secretin (+/-cholecystokinin [CCK]) causes a direct stimulation of the pancreas. Duodenal pancreatic secretions are then measured. The bicarbonate concentration should be > 80 mEq/L. CCK stimulates lipase, amylase, trypsin, and chymotrypsin which can also be measured.

Several breath tests for assessing pancreatic function are undergoing evaluation. Two of these are the cholesteryl-[14C]octanoate breath test and the HPLCN-benzoyl-tyrosyl-p-aminobenzoic acid/p-aminosalicylic acid (NBT-PABA/PAS) test. The results are very promising and may replace more invasive tests in the future.

Complications of Chronic Pancreatitis

A major complication is persistent and severe abdominal pain. In this setting
1) rule out continued ETOH use
2) rule out pseudocyst
3) an ERCP is warranted to define duct anatomy
4) can try high-dose pancreatic enzymes to shut of the enteropancreatic (intestine-pancreas) axis.

Pancreatic cancer develops in 4% of patients with chronic pancreatitis after 20 years.

Complications of chronic pancreatitis include gastric varices (from splenic vein thrombosis), B12 malabsorption, jaundice, pleural effusion, and brittle diabetes mellitus. The only skin involvement is tender red nodules from fat necrosis and this is uncommon.

The diabetes associated with chronic pancreatitis is different from the usual DM. It occurs when > 80% of the pancreas is destroyed. There is a decrease in production of insulin and glucagon. Because the pancreas is producing so little glucagon, the patient is very prone to hypoglycemia. Therefore, very loose control of the hyperglycemia is recommended. These patients do not have the retinopathy and nephropathy associated with the usual DM. They commonly have neuropathy but it is probably caused by alcoholism and/or malnutrition.

Treatment of Chronic Pancreatitis

Treatment includes pancreatic enzymes (20,000-30,000 units of lipase/day), decreasing dietary fat, and adding medium chain triglycerides to the diet. Pancreatic enzymes must either have an enteric coating or be given with antacids/H2 blockers because gastric acid destroys enzymes.

PANCREATIC NEOPLASMS

Pancreatic cancer [(pg 144, #430-431)] is fatal in 99% of patients no matter what the treatment modality. 80% of patients present with advanced disease. Heavy smokers have 2xN risk.

Classic presentation is weight loss, back pain, anorexia +/- diarrhea: Depending on the site and size of cancer, the patient may or may not have abdominal/back pain and may or may not have obstructive jaundice. Pain and weight loss are indicative of advanced disease. The pain typically has a gnawing quality, is not cured by eating, and occasionally radiates to the back. Chemotherapy and radiotherapy have not shown any benefit.

Treatment of pancreatic cancer. If the patient has a small pancreatic cancer + NO METS, then surgery is indicated (i.e., Whipple resection = pancreaticoduodenectomy). Pancreatic cancer WITH mets = no surgery; supportive (or experimental chemo) care only. You can put a stent in for biliary obstruction.

Glucagonoma is a glucagon-secreting alpha-cell tumor of the pancreas which causes a unique set of clinical findings. These are a very distinctive scaly necrolytic erythema, weight loss, anemia, and persistent hyperglycemia. Plasma glucagon (by RIA) is usually > 1000 pg/dl.

Insulinoma is a very rare insulin-secreting beta-cell tumor of the pancreas. This is covered in Endocrinology section (under Hypoglycemia).

Gastrinomas are discussed in the stomach section. Most (50%) are found in the duodenum, 24% in the pancreas. This diagnosis is likely when the serum gastrin > 500 and gastric acid present.

VIPomas are tumors which secrete vasoactive intestinal peptide (VIP). Two-thirds occur in the pancreas and over half of them are malignant. They cause a profuse secretory diarrhea ("pancreatic cholera"). Diagnosis: increased serum VIP level and hypokalemia.

BILIARY SYSTEM
CHOLELITHIASIS

Cholelithiasis is widespread—20% of women and 8% of men—and usually asymptomatic. It is not associated with hypercholesterolemia. The pathophysiology involves one or more of the following 3 factors:
1) Abnormal (lithogenic) bile secreted by the liver,
2) accelerated nucleation of microcrystals to macrocrystals, and
3) defective gall bladder emptying.

Cholelithiasis has been associated with obesity, oral contraceptive use, clofibrate treatment, and ileal disease or resection. 80% of bile stones are composed of radiolucent cholesterol and the remainder are of pigment.

Cholesterol stones: rapid weight loss in obese patient (prevented by aspirin or ursodeoxycholic acid), American Indians, octreotide use, ileal resection (Crohn disease).

Pigment stones: Clonorchis (biliary dwelling trematode), Sickle cell disease or anything else that causes hemolysis.

Diagnosis: Fatty food intolerance is a very nonspecific finding. To detect either the presence of stones or common duct obstruction, do an ultrasound (90% sensitive). If the ultrasound is technically inadequate, an oral cholecystogram can be done. Other procedures used for diagnosing common duct obstruction are ERCP and transhepatic cholangiography.

The HIDA scan (cholescintigraphy) is the best test for confirming acute cystic duct obstruction (i.e., acute cholecystitis) by imaging of the bile duct but not the gallbladder. [(pg 144, #432)]

Treatment of cholelithiasis: If the patient has gallstones and is symptomatic, do an elective cholecystectomy (or oral bile salts) as 70% of these patients have recurrence of the symptoms if not treated. If a patient has gallbladder stones but is asymptomatic, no treatment is indicated because only 20% subsequently develop symptoms.

Supplemental oral bile acid is "successful" in the treatment of cholesterol stones only; and only if the stones are < 1 cm, few in number, and if the patient is compliant—even so, the stones usually recur anyway! Not used much. There is no real role for lithotripsy.

Acalculous cholecystitis often occurs in seriously ill patients (e.g., major trauma, burns, after major surgeries). Diagnosis may be assisted by ultrasound or CT showing no stones but a large tense often thickened gallbladder with pericholecystic fluid (or no stones and a HIDA scan showing cystic duct obstruction). Treatment is cholecystectomy.

Common duct stones (choledocholithiasis) are removed by ERCP with prn endoscopic sphincterotomy. Think of this in the patient who persists in having RUQ pain after cholecystectomy or with symptoms of cholangitis (next) By the way, *choledochus* is a Latin term for *common bile duct*.

notes

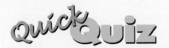

Cholangitis is a complication of common bile duct blockage. Nonsuppurative cholangitis is suggested by the triad of biliary colic, fever and chills, and jaundice (Charcot's triad). Suppurative cholangitis additionally has mental confusion, bacteremia, and septic shock. Antibiotics are indicated but are not sufficient treatment for suppurative cholangitis. When suppurative cholangitis is suspected, the best procedure for both diagnosis and treatment is ERCP with endoscopic sphincterotomy.

Emphysematous cholecystitis requires emergent laparotomy with cholecystectomy and antibiotics. In both suppurative cases, the antibiotics must be effective against both gram negative and anaerobic organisms. Do not use ceftriaxone—it can cause biliary concrements!

X-ray showing a gallbladder with a calcified outline ("porcelain gallbladder") suggests cancer and an open cholecystectomy is indicated.

PRIMARY BILIARY CIRRHOSIS

Primary Biliary Cirrhosis (PBC): Usually occurs in middle-aged women (pg 137, #409-410). The cause of PBC is unknown, but 70% have associated diseases of altered immunity (Sjögren, scleroderma, autoimmune thyroiditis, CREST) and the disease does run in families. 90% have a positive antimitochondrial antibody test (> 1:40) but the degree of elevation does not correlate with the severity of disease.

Symptoms: patients initially complain of itching—first in the palms and soles and later throughout the body. They later develop jaundice, hyperpigmentation, vitamin D de-pendent osteomalacia, and accelerated osteoporosis. They can get xanthomas and xanthelasmas from the hypercholesterolemia (but this does not convey increased risk of CAD because there is also an elevated HDL!). The disease is indolent, but relentlessly progressive. Symptomatic patients have a median survival of 10 years and asymptomatic patients live much longer. When the bilirubin > 2, the disease accelerates. Most die soon after the bilirubin reaches 10 unless liver transplantation is carried out.

Note: The antimitochondrial antibody test is the hallmark test for PBC. Even so, it is not a good indicator of the severity of PBC. The antimitochondrial antibody test is only occasionally positive in both autoimmune hepatitis and drug-induced chronic hepatitis; a high titer in a patient with autoimmune hepatitis suggests an overlap syndrome. (See Table 1-7)

Incidental discovery of a 2-5x increase in serum alkaline phosphatase has been the main stimulus for the increase in PBC diagnoses. Diagnosis is confirmed only with a liver biopsy showing granulomas. PBC patients also have a high hepatic copper level (but so do those with primary sclerosing cholangitis and Wilson disease).

Treatment: Ursodiol (ursodeoxycholate—a synthetic bile acid) is the best proven treatment available for PBC. It improves LFTs and decreases symptoms and it may retard (but not prevent) progression of the disease. Colchicine also helps to a lesser extent. Otherwise there is just symptomatic treatment. For pruritus: cholestyramine. For osteomalacia: Vit D, Estrogen, Calcium. For malabsorption: medium chain triglycerides and decrease dietary fat. Medical treatment has no effect on late disease.

For late disease, liver transplantation is the recommended procedure. It has been shown to significantly improve survival in late PBC. PBC is one of the most common disease indications for liver transplantation (hepatitis C is the most common)! To remember the main facts asked about this entity, think of the mitochondria in the liver being attacked by the anti-mitochondrial antibodies (an autoimmune problem like thyroiditis), thereby causing bile duct lesions and cirrhosis.

PRIMARY SCLEROSING CHOLANGITIS

Primary Sclerosing Cholangitis (PSC) has a strong association with colitis (75%!)—so it is mainly seen in ulcerative colitis but can be in Crohn disease involving the colon. Male:female is > 2:1. Unknown cause. Patients develop inflammation and

SEROLOGIC MARKERS IN PBC vs CAH	Primary Biliary Cirrhosis	Drug-induced CAH	Autoimmune CAH
Antimitochondrial Ab	90% Positive	occ Positive	occ Positive (low titers)
Anti-Smooth muscle Ab	Negative	Negative	Positive
Antinuclear Ab	usu Negative	Negative	Positive

Table 1-7: Serologic Markers in Primary Biliary Cirrhosis and Autoimmune Chronic Active Hepatitis

notes

sclerosis of the entire biliary tract (intra- & extrahepatic) leading to obstructive jaundice. Bilirubin and alkaline phosphatase levels are elevated (cholestatic pattern). There is an elevated hepatic copper level (as in primary biliary cirrhosis and Wilson disease) but the antimitochondrial antibody is negative. The total protein level gives an idea of how much the disease has affected liver function.

8-15% of PSC patients develop cholangiocarcinoma.

Patients are initially asymptomatic but eventually, with advanced disease, develop weakness and fatigue, itching, and jaundice.

Diagnosis of PSC is made with ERCP or transhepatic cholangiography. These reveal irregularly narrowed bile ducts with small bile duct ballooning just prior to obstructions producing the typical "beaded" appearance. With ERCP, if a dominant stricture exists, it can be dilated. Secondary causes of sclerosing cholangitis must be ruled out. These include: bacterial cholangitis (stones or bile-duct stricture), atypical anatomy (congenital or previous surgery), bile-duct neoplasms, and AIDS-associated cholangiopathy.

Treatment of PSC: The only sure treatment for PSC is a liver transplant; although colectomy cures ulcerative colitis, it does not change the course of this associated disease. High-dose ursodeoxycholic acid (20-25 mg/kg) may retard progression of disease.

Remember, when a patient presents with jaundice and increased alk phos and has history of chronic diarrhea or IBD, think of PSC!

LIVER

HEPATITIS NOTES

Hepatitis: Several notes: SGPT (ALT) is more liver-specific than SGOT (AST). To remember that ALT is the more liver specific, think of "L-L"; "ALT-Liver." With alcoholic hepatitis, the AST:ALT is about 3:1 because the alcohol damages mitochondria which are a source of AST. With viral hepatitis, the ALT is usually greater than the AST because its toxicity is more liver-specific. Note that Table 1-9 reviews the hepatitis serological tests.

HEPATITIS B

Hepatitis B: know the 3 main antigenic markers in hepatitis B—HBcAg, HBeAg, and HBsAg. See Table 1-8.

• HBsAg: There are 3 HBsAg+ proteins seen in the serum in patients with hepatitis B. One large, double shelled 42 nm particle that is the intact virion and two smaller 22 nm spherical or rod-shaped protein particles that outnumber the large particle up to 1000 to 1! These 22 nm HBsAg+ particles are thought to be just excess viral coat protein. The HBsAg has many different subtypes (adw, adr...) which have no clinical significance although they are used epidemiologically to evaluate outbreaks. Finding anti-HBs IgG in the serum indicates past exposure to either hepatitis B virion or to the vaccine.

• HBcAg+ protein is the core particle (inner shell) of the above 42 nm virion. This protein is retained in the hepatocyte until it is covered with HBsAg+ nucleocapsid outer shell which will then incorporate the DNA. Free HBcAg+ protein does not circulate in the serum. Antibody to HBcAg appears early in the disease (initially IgM, then IgG) and persists for life so anti-HBc IgG is the best marker for previous exposure to HBV.

• HBeAg is a soluble protein made from the same gene as HBcAg and, unlike HBcAg, HBeAg is secreted from the hepatocytes and circulated in the serum. It correlates with the quantity of intact virus and therefore with infectivity and liver inflammation. The HBe antibody (anti-HBe) appears several weeks after the illness. Detecting HBsAg and HBeAg indicated active virions and high infectivity (more so than HBsAg+ and HBeAg-). The tests for HBeAg and anti-HBe are often not available locally.

Hepatitis B is the only hepatitis virus composed of DNA. Incubation period is 1-6 months. It is transmitted by contaminated serum or blood products. Once infected, the first marker detectable in the serum is the antigen, HBsAg. This is followed by the appearance of antibody to the core antigen. After HBsAg becomes undetectable, there is a period of several weeks before the anti-HBs antibody becomes detectable. This is called the "window" and an anti-HBc IgM must be done during this period to confirm acute hepatitis B. See Figure 1-4 and Table 1-8.

Hepatitis B is strongly associated with polyarteritis nodosa (PAN). The surface antigen is found in 20-30% of these patients. It appears that the hepatitis B infection precipitates an autoimmune reaction resulting in PAN.

Clinical: First are prodromal constitutional symptoms which typically resolve at the time jaundice becomes apparent. Occasionally (10-15%) the prodromal symptoms are serum

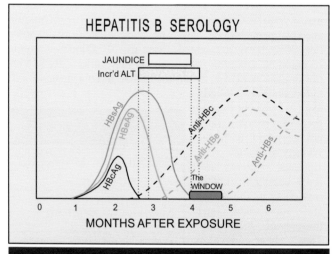

Figure 1-4: Hepatitis B serology vs. Time after Exposure

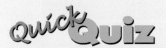

Quick Quiz

1) What are the alk phos, bilirubin, hepatic copper, and antimitochondrial antibody tests in PBC and PSC?

2) A patient presents with cholestatic jaundice and a history of IBD or chronic diarrhea. What do you think of? PBC or PSC? Why?

3) Regarding HBsAg, HBcAg, and HBeAg: Which is the best marker for infectivity? Which is the best marker for past infection?

4) What is the "window" period for Hepatitis B infection?

5) Polyarteritis nodosum is associated with which hepatitis virus?

6) Are hepatitis B vaccines safe for pregnant patients?

7) How would you confirm that hepatitis B vaccine was immunogenic?

8) Know the scenarios!

sickness-like with fever, arthritis, urticaria, and angioedema. This seems to be caused by circulating immune complexes (especially HBsAg+ anti-HBs) activating the complement system. With the onset of jaundice, the patient usually feels much better but may have liver swelling and tenderness and cholestatic symptoms.

Removal of HBV is T cell mediated and the only purpose of anti-HBsAg is to prevent reinfection.

Hepatitis B immune globulin (HBIG; anti-HBs) provides some protection against hepatitis B, although it appears to only decrease the severity of illness rather than protect the patient from disease. It is effective as prophylaxis and when given in early infection.

The two hepatitis B vaccines are composed of HBsAg. They are equally effective and they are safe for pregnant patients. It is best if the hepatitis B vaccine is given before the patient is exposed to HBV. 95% of immunocompetent patients develop antibodies whereas only about 50% of dialysis patients do. Because these vaccines are surface antigens, to ensure effectiveness after the course of vaccine has been given, check for anti-HBs—there will be no anti-HBc.

The likelihood of developing chronic HBV is inversely related to age. Chronic HBV occurs in 90% of infants infected at birth, 25-50% in children age 1-5 yrs, and 5% in older children and adults. There is now universal preschool vaccination in the US. Overall, less than 1% of patients with hepatitis B develop fulminant hepatitis, but about 5-7% develop chronic carrier states. There are 3 types of carrier states:

1) asymptomatic

2) chronic persistent hepatitis and

3) chronic hepatitis B. 1 & 2 are benign.

A liver biopsy is required to differentiate 2 & 3. Chronic hepatitis B is a serious illness—it often progresses to cirrhosis and is strongly associated with hepatocellular cancer [pg 142, #424]. Poor results with liver transplantation so far—not considered an indication.

Scenarios:

• A newborn of a mother with hepatitis B should be given HBIG and hepatitis B vaccination. There is a 5-10% transplacental transmission of HBV.

• If an asymptomatic patient has HBsAg in the serum, it means either the patient is a carrier or the patient has early hepatitis B—so initial action is only to follow closely (once the patient is infected, neither vaccine nor HBIG helps).

• If a person has possible blood exposure to a person with an acute HBV infection and the HBsAg is still negative, the CDC recommends giving that person hepatitis B immune globulin (HBIG) followed by a complete course of HBV vaccinations. The HBIG alone is to be given to the sexual contacts of carriers and to the household contacts of patients with acute infection if there is no known blood exposure. If there is suspected blood exposure, check the HBsAg and, if negative, give the vaccine in addition to the HBIG. This goes the same for a pregnant patient.

Note: several months after an episode of hepatitis B, check for loss of HBsAg and HBV-DNA to ensure that it has not become chronic.

Know the hepatitis B scenarios ! (including those in Table 1-8)

Table 1-8: Interpretation of Hepatitis B tests			
HEPATITIS B SCENARIOS			
HBsAg	HBcAb	HBsAb	Interpretation
+	–	–	Acute Infection
+	+	–	3 poss: 1) Acute Infection 2) Chronic Hep B (high AST) 3) Carrier (normal enzymes)
–	–	+	2 poss: 1) Remote infection 2) Immunized
–	+	+	Remote infection
–	+	–	3 poss: 1) Window disease 2) Remote infection 3) False positive
+	+	+	More than 1 infection. E.g., IV drug user or renal dialysis patient with both acute and chronic hepatitis B.

TYPES OF VIRAL HEPATITIS AND THEIR SEROLOGICAL TEST								
	Anti-HAV IgM	Anti-HAV IgG	HBsAg	Anti-HBs IgM	Anti-HBs IgG	Anti-HBc IgM	Anti-HBc IgG	HBeAg	Anti-HDV
Acute Hepatitis A	+	-	-						
Previous HAV	-	+	-						
Acute HBV	-		+early	+late	-	+	-	+	-
Acute HBV - window			-	-	-	+	-	-	-
Chronic active HBV			15%	-	rarely	-	+	usu +	-
Remote HBV			-	-	+	-	+	-	-
Immunized - HBV			-	-	+	-	-	-	-
Acute Hepatitis D - (w acute HB)			+early	+late	-	+	-	+	+
Acute Hepatitis D - (w CAH)			15%	-	rarely	-	+	usu +	+

Table 1-9: Hepatitis and Serological Test

HEPATITIS A

Hepatitis A is an RNA virus. It is easily transmitted fecal-orally—usually via food or water. It can be sexually transmitted. There is no transplacental transmission! There are no carrier or persistent states although occasionally they get prolonged cholestasis (with increased bili and alk phos) for up to 4 months. Incubation period is 15-50 days.

Diagnosis of acute infection: high titers of anti-HAV IgM in serum (IgG only indicates a previous infection). Symptoms are unusual in children and very common in adults (70%). Complications are rare—about 1% chance of fulminant hepatitis. Immune globulin (IG) is good prophylaxis only against HAV (use HBIG for hepatitis B). (See Figure 1-5)

An inactivated hepatitis A vaccine (Havrix and Vaqta) is available. It is for use in patients 2 years or older and given as 2 doses, 6 months apart. Virtually all those completing the series develop protective levels of antibody to hepatitis A virus (anti-HAV). Trends based on what is now known of the antibody levels suggest protection for up to 20 years in those who complete the series.

Indications for use of HAV vaccine:
• high risk behavior,
• children > 2 years old in communities with high rates,
• chronic liver disease,
• travel in high risk countries.
• HAV vaccine is also given to all patients with hepatitis C; if these patients get hepatitis A, it can be fulminant.

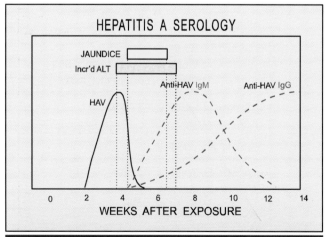

HEPATITIS A SEROLOGY

JAUNDICE
Incr'd ALT
Anti-HAV IgM
Anti-HAV IgG
HAV

0   2   4   6   8   10   12   14
WEEKS AFTER EXPOSURE

Figure 1-5: Hepatitis A serology vs. Time after Exposure

HEPATITIS C

Hepatitis C—single strand RNA virus. It is now the most common liver disease in the U.S. (know this section well!). Hepatitis C has blood-borne transmission and had been the cause of 90% of transfusion-associated hepatitis prior to the 1990s. Since then, especially with the 2nd generation anti-HCV assays, the incidence of HCV-related hepatitis has become very rare. Most HCV infections in the U.S. are genotype 1 which happens to be less responsive to treatment.

Those at increased risk for hepatitis C:
1) Especially IV drug abusers; common in prisons
2) High risk sexual behavior: with STD, sex with prostitutes, > 5 sexual partners per year
3) Blood transfusion before 1990
4) Tattoos, Body piercing
5) Snorting cocaine

Whereas only 1% of adults with hepatitis B develop chronic disease, 70-80% of acute HCV infections become chronic!

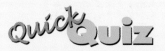

1) How common is chronic hepatitis in hepatitis C infection? In hepatitis A infection?

2) With what coinfection can hepatitis A become fulminant?

3) Which hepatitis infection is mixed cryoglobulinemia strongly associated? How does it present?

4) What test ensures that a hepatitis C infection did not become chronic?

5) Which virus does hepatitis D require to replicate?

6) Hepatitis E is associated with which risk factor?

7) What test is the most specific test for type 1 autoimmune hepatitis?

Hepatitis B has high virus counts whereas hepatitis C has <u>low</u> virus counts. These low virus counts are consistent with the more insidious nature of hepatitis C:

• Only 25% of acute infections are symptomatic
• HCV infection has an increased likelihood to become chronic
• For the chronic form to be relatively benign (25% are only carriers, 50% have no symptoms but have abnormal LFTs, 25% have chronic active disease with symptoms).
• It is also consistent with the low rates of sexual transmission seen in monogamous couples—5% after 10-20 years! This is low but it does occur—so safe sex is required! Sexual transmission increases with multiple sexual partners.
• Needle stick transmission from a known infected patient is 5-10%.
• Transplacental infection: < 5 %—although this is only a little less than hepatitis B (5-10%).

Extrahepatic disease includes small vessel vasculitis with glomerulonephritis and neuropathy, mixed cryoglobulinemia, and porphyria cutanea tarda. Mixed cryoglobulinemia presents as a small vessel (leukocytoclastic) vasculitis with a rash consisting of "palpable purpura" or "crops of purple papules".

70-80% of patients infected with HCV develop chronic hepatitis—and about 25% of these get end-stage cirrhosis after 20-25 years! And 1-4% of patients with cirrhosis develop hepatoma each year. Chronic HCV infection has become the #1 cause of liver transplants in the US.

Patients with high risk behavior presenting with probable hepatitis C who have negative hepatitis B tests are still given HBIG with the hepatitis vaccine because the combination of hepatitis B and hepatitis C is extremely severe and often fatal. There is no vaccine for hepatitis C although it appears there will be one in a few years.

Tests:

• Within 2-4 months after an episode of hepatitis C, recheck for loss of HCV-RNA (PCR) to ensure that it has not become chronic. Note that this HCV-RNA test is not quantitative—but it is sensitive and can determine if there are more than 1,000 HCV equivalents/ml.
• In a person positive for anti-HCV, confirm positive antibody with the RIBA test (to exclude false positive test). If the RIBA is positive, check for active virus with HCV-RNA. This is necessary because the anti-HCV does not confer immunity (as does the HBV antibody).

Mixed cryoglobulinemia can result from chronic hepatitis B or C (in addition to various other occult viral, bacterial, and fungal infections).

HEPATITIS D

Hepatitis D is an RNA virus which requires a coexistent hepatitis B virus infection for the hepatitis D to become pathogenic. It is usually found in IV drug abusers and high-risk HBsAg carriers. It usually does not make an acute HBV infection much worse but, if acquired as a superinfection in an HBV carrier, the infection is frequently very severe. If acquired acutely, HDV does not increase risk of chronic hepatitis B. Immunity to hepatitis B implies immunity to hepatitis D. Diagnosis: Anti-HDV IgM.

HEPATITIS E

Hepatitis E—single strand RNA virus. Fecal/oral spread like HAV. Found in the Far East, Africa, and Central America. Usually due to contamination of water supplies after monsoon flooding. Like hepatitis A, no chronic form is known. Unlike hepatitis A, hepatitis E carries a very high risk for fulminant hepatitis in the third trimester of pregnancy—with a 20% fatality rate. With acute hepatitis in a traveler and negative serology, think of Hepatitis E.

HEPATITIS G

Hepatitis G is blood-borne like hepatitis B and C. Mode of transmission is not well defined but is similar to HCV. There is evidence of infection in 1.5% of blood donors. It causes < 0.5% of community-acquired hepatitis. There is no evidence that HGV causes chronic liver disease.

CHRONIC HEPATITIS

Autoimmune Chronic Hepatitis

Autoimmune: Type 1 autoimmune hepatitis usually has an insidious onset and is most often found in young women. Type 2 is a childhood disease and will not be discussed. 50% of adult patients with autoimmune chronic hepatitis also have other disorders of altered immunity—thyroiditis, Coombs+ anemia, and ITP. Autoantibodies are common; affected patients often have a positive ANA, anti-dsDNA, smooth muscle antibody (SMA), ANCA, and anti-actin. The SMA test is the most specific of the autoantibody tests for type 1 and it is positive in about 80% of patients with type 1 autoimmune hepatitis (see Table 1-7). It is occasionally seen as an overlap syndrome with PBC or PSC.

Early diagnosis is essential because this form of chronic hepatitis responds well to treatment. Other forms of hepatitis must be excluded and the following autoantibody tests are done: ANA, SMA, ANCA. Antimitochondrial antibody may also be done—it is only occasionally slightly positive but high titer occurs in primary biliary cirrhosis and indicates an overlap syndrome. Diagnosis is confirmed by characteristic changes being found on histologic examination of a liver biopsy. These changes are characteristic but not specific, so drug history and serologic tests are required to rule out other types of hepatitis.

Treatment. Unlike other types of hepatitis, patients with autoimmune chronic hepatitis usually have a rapid reversal of symptoms and increased survival with prednisone +/- azathioprine. Azathioprine is used as a steroid-sparing drug—alone it has no effect. Alpha interferon, although used in chronic hepatitis B&C, exacerbates autoimmune hepatitis and is therefore contraindicated. Despite the response to the above treatment, there is no cure for autoimmune hepatitis and it frequently progresses to cirrhosis and sometimes hepatocellular carcinoma (less often than with viral chronic hepatitis). Liver transplant is indicated for end-stage disease, although the disease process will slowly recur.

Chronic Viral Hepatitis

Chronic hepatitis **B**: Eventually leads to cirrhosis. There is a high risk of hepatocellular cancer, 6% annually in cirrhotics. Medications used to treat are alpha-interferon and lamivudine. Alpha-interferon results in a 35% complete remission and infrequent relapse. Lamivudine can also suppress chronic hepatitis B but only infrequently causes loss of HBV-DNA.

Chronic hepatitis **C**: Also eventually leads to cirrhosis. There is also a high risk of hepatocellular cancer, 7% annually in cirrhotics. Medications used to treat are alpha-interferon and ribavirin. A 6-month course of alpha-interferon induces a treatment response in 30-40% but there is only a 15% sustained loss of HCV-RNA (much worse than with hepatitis B). Longer duration of therapy is being evaluated. Combination interferon-ribavirin therapy for 12 months results in a 35-45% loss of HCV-RNA. See the acute forms discussed previously for more on these diseases.

Treatment with alpha-interferon (+/- ribavirin) significantly reduces the risk of hepatocellular cancer in those with chronic hepatitis C but NOT those with chronic hepatitis B.

Again note: Several months after an episode of hepatitis C, recheck for loss of HCV-RNA to ensure that it has not become chronic. After hepatitis B, check to ensure loss of HBsAg and HBV-DNA.

Drug-related Chronic Hepatitis

Drug-related chronic hepatitis is associated with methyldopa, acetaminophen, trazodone, nitrofurantoin, phenytoin [pg 135, #405], and INH (although INH far more commonly causes an acute hepatitis). Histologic changes are similar to autoimmune hepatitis and the patients are often ANA +. Hypergammaglobulinemia is also often present. Best treatment is to stop the drug.

Drug-related liver disease (acute) can be caused by both the direct toxic, allergic, and/or the idiosyncratic effects of drugs. Acetaminophen causes a direct toxic effect. Drugs causing an idiosyncratic effect are: halothane, phenytoin, chlorpromazine, and erythromycin. Drugs causing both toxic and idiopathic effects: methyldopa, INH (isoniazid), and sodium valproate.

Birth control pills, anabolic steroids, chlorpromazine and erythromycin are associated with cholestasis but not hepatitis.

Expansion on INH, oral contraceptives, acetaminophen, and alcohol:

Acetaminophen poisoning is discussed in the Poisoning section of General IM. Briefly: When acetaminophen is ingested, 90% of it is processed via the glucuronidation pathway, 5% is excreted unchanged in the urine, and 5% is oxidized by the cytochrome P-450 system. The P-450 system produces a toxic intermediate compound (N-acetyl-*p*-benzoquinoneimine, NAPQI) which is quickly reduced by glutathione. When there is an acetaminophen overdose, glutathione is rapidly depleted and the resulting unreduced toxin causes direct liver damage.

Alcohol-acetaminophen syndrome. Chronic moderate-to-heavy use of alcohol has a two-fold effect: the cytochrome P-450 system is cranked up (i.e., more NAPQI is produced) and the amount of glutathione is decreased (so less is available for detoxifying the NAPQI). Therefore long-time users of moderate to heavy amounts of alcohol who take acetaminophen in normal or higher doses are at-risk for severe hepatic toxicity or liver failure.

Glutathione levels are depressed in malnutrition. Acetaminophen liver toxicity also may develop by not eating for 3-4 days with an acute viral illness and taking therapeutic doses of acetaminophen (i.e., < 4.0 gm/d)!!

Again: Know that acetaminophen liver damage is potentiated with chronic alcohol use, heavy alcohol use, malnutrition, and even dieting.

Alcoholic liver disease results in a macrovesicular fat accumulation—as also seen in obesity, AODM, protein malnutrition, prolonged IV hyperalimentation, and drugs (mentioned in the next paragraph). There is also a PMN infiltration in the liver. Women are more susceptible to alcoholic liver disease than men. Alcohol induces GGT so this enzyme is disproportionately high in alcoholic liver disease. Usually there is a discordance between SGOT (AST) and SGPT (ALT) in this disease, with an AST:ALT ratio of 3:1. The AST is virtually always less than 300—even with severe alcoholic liver injury.

There are several other drugs which cause macrovesicular fat accumulations similar to alcoholic hepatitis. These include amiodarone and corticosteroids.

Methotrexate can cause an indolent asymptomatic liver disease which progresses to cirrhosis.

notes

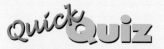

1) What is the treatment of autoimmune chronic hepatitis?

2) What is the risk of cirrhosis and liver cancer with chronic active hepatitis B? With C?

3) What is the alcohol-acetaminophen syndrome?

4) How are glutathione levels associated with acetaminophen toxicity?

5) What disease is most probable in a patient with tender hepatomegaly, a RUQ bruit, bloody ascites, a high alkaline phosphatase and a very elevated alpha-fetoprotein level?

6) Name all the causes of cirrhosis.

7) Bleeding of esophageal varices is best correlated with what aspect of the varices?

8) What drug is associated with decreased rebleeds?

INH causes an occasional mild, transient increase in liver enzymes. 1% of these develop a more severe hepatitis—the severity of which correlates with age.

Oral contraceptives are associated with benign hepatic adenoma, peliosis hepatis (blood filled sinusoids), and focal nodular hyperplasia of the liver.

Direct toxic effect is modified by other factors—nutrition etc. Toxic effects may be additive. Alcoholics are very susceptible to acetaminophen liver damage because alcohol induces the cytochrome P-450 system (in most questions, acetaminophen is presented as an "over the counter pain reliever"). The combination may cause fulminant hepatitis.

Reye syndrome occurs exclusively in children < 15 years old. Although rare, it tends to occur after a recent viral illness, especially influenza A or B or varicella (chicken pox), and especially when there has been concurrent ASA use. These patients get a fatty liver (microvesicular—as in acute fatty liver of pregnancy) and progressive encephalopathy. Elevated ALT, AST, NH_3, and prothrombin time. Hypoglycemia, as a result of severe liver failure, is common. There is a 50% mortality.

Etceteras...

Etc.: As mentioned, other causes of chronic hepatitis are alcohol, alpha-1-antitrypsin deficiency, Wilson disease, and hemochromatosis. Corticosteroids and pentoxifylline are of transient benefit in severe alcoholic hepatitis.

HEPATOCELLULAR CANCER

Hepatocellular cancer (hepatoma). 75% have antecedent cirrhosis. Hepatomas are associated with chronic liver disease of any type: chronic hepatitis B & C, hemochromatosis, alpha-1 antitrypsin deficiency, alcoholic liver disease, and autoimmune hepatitis. In addition, hepatomas are associated with aflatoxin (raw peanuts or raw peanut butter). Alcoholic liver disease is the most common cause of hepatomas in the US. Chronic hepatitis B infection acquired at birth is the most common cause in developing countries.

Hepatoma is associated with tender hepatomegaly, a bruit in RUQ, bloody ascites, high alkaline phosphatase, and 70-80% have a very elevated alpha-fetoprotein level.

Hypercalcemia and high hematocrit levels are indications of hepatoma-associated paraneoplastic syndromes and are clues to the diagnosis. Think of hepatocellular cancer in any cirrhotic who decompensates without an obvious reason.

Remember that alpha-interferon treatment in chronic hepatitis C reduces the risk of hepatoma.

CIRRHOSIS

Overview

Causes of Cirrhosis: alcohol (most common cause in U.S.: [pg 136, #407; pg 138, #412-413; pg 139, #415-417]), hepatitis (B or C), postnecrotic (drugs and toxins), biliary disease, cardiac (from severe, prolonged right-sided CHF—which is rare), alpha-1 antitrypsin deficiency, hemochromatosis, Wilson disease, and schistosomiasis.

Complications of Cirrhosis

Esophageal variceal hemorrhage: One third of patients with esophageal varices bleed and each bleed carries 1/3 mortality. With a bleed, wedged:free portal pressure gradient is usually > 12 mmHg (normal ≤ 6), but chance of bleeding better correlates with the size of the varices.

Primary therapy of bleeding varices is endoscopic sclerotherapy or banding. "TIPS" is used for cases that rebleed. TIPS = transjugular intrahepatic portal systemic shunt. Sclerotherapy is not good prophylaxis against the first hemorrhage—it actually appears to make things worse.

Trials on vasoconstrictive therapy have been inconclusive. The best therapy appears to be IV infusion of somatostatin or its analogue, octreotide which are splanchnic vasoconstrictors. Vasopressin with simultaneous nitroglycerin (to minimize the vasoconstrictive side-effect of vasopressin) has been used but is associated with more complications.

The Sengstaken-Blakemore tube is rarely used anymore because it has a high rate of complications.

Propranolol, with or without isosorbide dinitrate decreases rebleeds and may delay or prevent the occurrence of the first variceal bleed. For illustrations of varices: [pg 140, #418-420].

Ascites is discussed in the next section

notes

Hepatic encephalopathy may be precipitated by:
- GI bleed,
- infections (pneumonia, bacteremia, urosepsis, and sponta-neous bacterial peritonitis—SBP),
- increased dietary protein • constipation
- hypokalemia, • sedatives,
- tranquilizers, • azotemia
- alkalosis which increases ammonia/ammonium ratio (NH_3/NH_4^+)—as only the non-ionized form, NH_3 (ammo-nia), crosses the blood-brain barrier.

Acidosis has the opposite effect. Signs of hepatic encephalopa-thy include fetor hepaticus (unique musty odor to breath and urine), hyperreflexia, and asterixis. Treat with dietary protein restriction and lactulose—this disaccharide is broken down by colonic bacteria, thereby acidifying the colon contents and keeping the NH_4^+ content high.

Hepatorenal syndrome is also called "oliguric hepatic failure." The renal failure is caused by renal vasoconstriction during severe, decompensated cirrhosis. Usually fatal. Frequently iatrogenic—secondary to diuretics, NSAIDs, aminoglyco-sides, IV contrast, and paracentesis.

Again note: alcohol causes malabsorption of some vitamins including vitamin K—so, if the prothrombin time in an alco-holic is prolonged and is easily corrected by IM vitamin K, then it is probably due to malabsorption—not liver disease (which affects more of the coagulation factors and is there-fore harder to correct).

ASCITES

Ascites. Determining the cause of ascites often requires analy-sis of a peritoneal tap specimen for appearance, cell count with differential, cytology, total protein, and albumin.
Appearance: bloody suggests a tumor; cloudy—an infection; milky—lymphatic obstruction.
Cell count: If the cell count is elevated, a C&S is done.
  Chemistry: Portal hypertension is indicated by a serum-to-ascites albumin gradient (SAAG) >1.1 g/dL (i.e., low level

---

of albumin in the ascites) and is seen in ascites due to RHF, cirrhosis, fulminant liver failure, Budd-Chiari syndrome [pg 141, #421], and myxedema. A SAAG < 1.1 (i.e., high level of albumin in the ascites and no portal HTN) is seen with as-cites due to tuberculosis peritonitis, nephrotic syndrome, pancreatitis, and peritoneal carcinomatosis.
An elevated ascites protein level (≥ 2.5) is seen in all cases that cause increased levels of albumin. It is also seen in cardiac ascites! (See Table 1-10)

Cirrhosis-induced ascites: Ascitic fluid is resorbed via the peri-toneal surface. Maximum capacity is about 900 cc/d. So if you try to diurese off > 1 liter/d, it is at the expense of in-travascular volume. This disease causes the most avid so-dium retention state known.
Note that a chylous ascites is due to lymph blockage (trauma, tumors, TB, and filariasis), not cirrhosis or CHF. In cir-rhotics, when the protein level in the fluid is < 1.0, there is decreased opsonic activity, and spontaneous bacterial perito-nitis is more likely to develop. Peritonitis is indicated by a peritoneal fluid with > 250 PMN/cc. Usual causes are E. coli, then S. pneumoniae, then Klebsiella.

Treatment: mainly Na^+ and water restriction—1 gm Na^+ (= 2 gm salt) and 2,000 cc water. Then, if needed, start spiro-nolactone, then a loop diuretic. Stop all anti-prostaglandin medications (ASA...) because these decrease urinary Na^+ ex-cretion! Also do not give an aminoglycoside in this setting as it may precipitate renal failure. Again, do not diurese > 1 li-ter/d. It is okay to do daily paracenteses (up to 4 liters/d) dur-ing the initial treatment of recent onset ascites or with severe refractory ascites **IF** the patient's renal function is normal. Albumin is also indicated in life-threatening ascites **although** it has only a short-term effect. Peritoneovenous shunt use is limited by shunt failure and increased variceal bleeding.

HEREDITARY LIVER DISEASE

Review of Bilirubin

Review of bilirubin. Hyperbilirubinuria is the main finding in hereditary liver diseases. In general, only conjugated bilirubin passes the glomeruli and is excreted in the urine. The unconjugated bilirubin is tightly bound to albumin and this complex is too large to pass through the glomerulus. Conjugated bilirubin is less tightly bound to albumin and the 5% unbound portion easily passes into the urine. So—bilirubinuria means conjugated hyperbilirubinemia. Because bilirubin is conjugated in the liver, bilirubinuria is an indica-tion of cholestasis.

...with UNCONJUGATED bilirubin

Gilbert syndrome is a very common, benign, chronic disor-der resulting in a mild, unconjugated hyperbilirubinemia. Remember: unconjugated = indirect = without bilirubinuria. The jaundice comes and goes and is brought on by physical stress (especially surgery, exertion, and infection), fasting, and alcohol ingestion. About 7% of the population has Gil-

---

Table 1-10: Causes of Ascites and the Associated Findings		
PROTEIN AND ALBUMIN IN ASCITES		
CAUSES	Serum/Ascites albumin	Ascites T. protein
Cirrhosis, Liver failure, Budd-Chiari synd, myxedema, and SBP	> 1.1	< 2.5
Right heart failure	> 1.1	> 2.5
TB peritonitis, nephrotic synd, pancreatitis, and Peritoneal carcinomatosis	< 1.1	> 2.5

notes

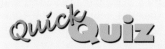

bert syndrome. It appears to be an autosomal dominant syndrome with variable penetrance! It is due to decreased or absent glucuronyl transferase in the liver cells. Half of patients have a very low grade chronic hemolysis. This probably reflects two separate syndromes but, for now, they are still grouped together. Phenobarbital stimulates glucuronyl transferase and decreases the bilirubin level. Diagnosis: Increased unconjugated bilirubin after prolonged fasting. No treatment is needed.

Crigler-Najjar syndrome causes a moderate (type II) to severe (type I) unconjugated (indirect) hyperbilirubinemia. Rare. Similar in etiology to Gilbert syndrome, it is due to decreased (II) or absent (I) glucuronyl transferase in the liver cells.

...with CONJUGATED bilirubin

Dubin-Johnson syndrome—conjugated hyperbilirubinemia (although some unconjugated). Rotor syndrome is a variant of Dubin-Johnson also with conjugated hyperbilirubinemia. The difference between them is that Rotor syndrome does not have the pigment granules in the centrilobular hepatocytes which are seen in Dubin-Johnson syndrome.

Note: If a patient is noted to have increased conjugated bilirubin after a major surgery, it is not Gilbert syndrome (which is unconjugated). It is most likely an entity called benign postoperative cholestasis. This is most often seen if the patient became hypotensive or required many transfusions during the operation.

Alpha1-antitrypsin deficiency

Alpha$_1$-antitrypsin deficiency (autosomal recessive) causes a chronic hepatitis eventually leading to cirrhosis. Diagnose with electrophoresis. Treatment: liver transplant—it does not recur in the transplanted liver!

Hemochromatosis

Hemochromatosis—two types—genetic and acquired. The acquired form is usually from a chronic anemia with $2°$ erythropoiesis such as sideroblastic anemia or thalassemia. The genetic form is autosomal recessive (AR). In both types, there

there is abnormally increased intestinal iron absorption which leads to iron deposition in the tissues. This iron deposition causes fibrosis and damage to organs—especially the liver, heart, pancreas, and pituitary. Clinical:
- hepatomegaly (95%),
- gray hyperpigmentation (90%) [pg 137, #411],
- secondary diabetes (65%),
- arthropathy (40%-esp 2nd and 3rd MCP joints), and
- cardiac involvement (15%).

Secondary hypogonadism also occurs and is caused by depression of the hypothalamic-pituitary axis. There is a 25-30% risk for hepatocellular cancer in patients with cirrhosis caused by this disease—higher than any other cause!

Diagnosis of hemochromatosis is suggested by high levels of serum Fe, ferritin, and transferrin levels. The most helpful screening test is transferrin saturation > 45%. Liver biopsy confirms the diagnosis. But, if this disease is successfully treated early enough—especially if cirrhosis is not present—patients have a normal life span with negligible risk of cancer. Initial treatment is weekly phlebotomies. This results in decreased skin pigmentation, improved cardiac function, and prolonged life expectancy. But if already lost, the secondary sex characteristics do not return (the damage is done!). Note that symptomatic hemochromatosis is 10x more frequent in men—this is probably because of the effect menses has on iron stores in women.

Wilson Disease

Wilson disease is an autosomal recessive disorder which usually presents as liver disease or neurologic/psychiatric dysfunction in adolescents. It usually presents between ages 15-25. Other symptoms include arthritis from chondrocalcinosis. Wilson disease is caused by impaired excretion of copper into bile which results in an excess copper in body tissues—especially the liver. Hemolysis is common. Serum ceruloplasmin is low (in most liver diseases it is high) and urinary copper level is high. Kayser-Fleischer rings are pathognomonic [pg 141, #422]. These consist of a single brownish corneal ring, formed by copper depositing along the outer edge of the cornea. Liver biopsy confirms the diagnosis; it shows a high liver copper level (but remember, so does PBC and PSC!). Treatment: Chelation with penicillamine (must give supplemental pyridoxine with this drug). If the patient cannot tolerate penicillamine or has progressive neurologic manifestations, trientine is used. Zinc salts are a third option. Patients may be maintained indefinitely on penicillamine or trientine. A liver transplant cures Wilson disease!

In fulminant Wilson disease, there is severe hemolytic anemia and high serum copper level due to the release of copper from the liver. Penicillamine therapy is not effective; the only treatment is liver transplant.

Fatty Liver of Pregnancy

Fatty liver of pregnancy is a very serious condition in which there is microvesicular fat deposition in the liver (as in Reye syndrome). It occurs in the last trimester and associated with encephalopathy, hypoglycemia (again like Reye syndrome)

notes

preeclampsia, pancreatitis, DIC, and renal failure. Early delivery is required.

LIVER TRANSPLANT

Liver transplant (know!) is considered for almost all patients with irreversible end-stage acute and chronic liver disease. The selection process excludes many of these. The selection is usually made by a liver transplant committee at the liver transplant center. The process is inexact and the waiting period for a liver is often over a year. Patients with chronic, progressive liver disease should be evaluated early in the course of the disease.

The recently released Model for End-stage Liver Disease (MELD) scale gives a fairly accurate short-term (3-6 month) prediction of mortality risk and is used to determine organ allocation for liver transplant. It uses bilirubin and creatinine levels, INR (normalized prothrombin time), and etiology of liver disease in its calculation. The MELD score is:

$$3.8\log_e(\text{bilirubin [mg/dL]}) + 11.2\log_e(\text{INR}) + 9.6\log_e(\text{creatinine [mg/dL]}) + 6.4(\text{etiology})$$
where etiology = 0 if cholestatic or alcoholic, 1 otherwise

Common indications for liver transplant: most types of chronic end-stage liver disease, metabolic liver disease, unresectable confined liver cancer, primary and secondary biliary cirrhosis, primary sclerosing cholangitis, and fulminant hepatitis.

Associated biochemical indications seen in end-stage chronic liver disease are bilirubin 10-15 mg/dl, albumin < 2.5, and a PT > 3-5 sec. Other signs/symptoms suggesting it is time to transplant: intractable pruritus, hepatic encephalopathy, bacterial peritonitis, intractable ascites, and the development of hepatocellular carcinoma.

Controversial: using liver transplant to treat alcoholic cirrhosis, chronic hepatitis B, and primary hepatocellular malignancies.

Absolute contraindications: preexisting advanced or uncontrolled non-hepatic disease, active alcohol or drug abuse, life-threatening systemic disease, metastatic cancer, and HIV infection. There are many relative contraindications including advanced age.

NUTRITION

VITAMIN DEFICIENCIES

Time until onset of symptoms of vitamin or mineral deficiency—as when on TPN without vitamin supplementation (and barring other problems) know!:

Weeks: Water soluble vitamins, magnesium (muscle stiffness and cramps—often causes tetany in patients with Crohn disease), zinc (acrodermatitis and poor wound healing), and essential fatty acids.

Months: Cu (hypochromic, microcytic anemia), and vitamin K (bleeding, high PT).

Year: Vitamin A & D (below), selenium (myalgias, cardiomyopathy, and hemolytic anemia), and chromium (glucose intolerance and peripheral neuropathy).

Several years: Iron, cobalt (anemia).

Many years: B12

These deficiencies are important; know them cold! A good way to review this section is to fill in the following sentence, using the appropriate times, symptoms, and mineral deficiencies from above.

If, after 1-2 (____), a patient on TPN develops (____), you would suspect (____).

More on vitamin deficiencies. Vitamins B and C are water soluble while vitamins A, D, E, and K are lipid soluble. These will be discussed in this order. Know all about vitamins and minerals!

Vitamin B1 is thiamine. Thiamine deficiency causes beriberi. It usually develops in alcoholics or in patients on chronic dialysis. There are two major manifestations of thiamine deficiency: wet beriberi and dry beriberi.

Wet beriberi: Symptoms of wet beriberi are heart failure, ascites, peripheral edema, and often an accompanying peripheral edema.

Dry beriberi: is confined to the nervous system (central and peripheral): peripheral neuropathy (symmetrical sensory, motor, and reflex loss), Wernicke encephalopathy (vomiting and nystagmus, ophthalmoplegia, ataxia, and mental deterioration), and Korsakoff syndrome (confabulation, retrograde amnesia). Korsakoff syndrome can be thought of as late stage Wernicke encephalopathy. Thiamine replacement usually cures Wernicke encephalopathy but it only reverses symptoms in half of patients with Korsakoff syndrome.

Vitamin B2 is riboflavin. B2 deficiency almost invariably occurs in association with other vitamin deficiencies. Phenothiazines and tricyclic antidepressants increase the tendency to develop riboflavin deficiency. Patients present with a normochromic normocytic anemia, sore throat with hyperemic mucosa and glossitis, cheilosis, angular stomatitis, and a seborrheic dermatitis especially involving the perineal/scrotal area. Symptoms are reversed with riboflavin.

Vitamin B6 is pyridoxine. Deficiency is rare and usually caused by drugs but may also be seen with general malabsorption syndromes and chronic alcoholism. The main drug culprits are INH, cycloserine, and penicillamine. Presenting symptoms include glossitis, cheilosis, vomiting, and seizures.

Vitamin B12 deficiency is discussed in the Hematology section. It results in a macrocytic anemia, smooth tongue, and subacute combined degeneration of the spinal cord.

Niacin deficiency causes pellagra. Niacin (nicotinic acid) is made from tryptophan in the body (so it is not actually a "vitamin"). Niacin deficiency is rare in the U.S. because niacin is now added to grains. It is still seen in carcinoid syndrome, in which tryptophan is used up, and when isoniazid is used in

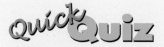

treating TB. Presenting signs of niacin deficiency are a dermatitis—especially on sun-exposed surfaces, glossitis ("bald tongue"), stomatitis, proctitis, diarrhea, and changing mental status ranging from depression to dementia to psychosis (remember these by the 3 Ds-mucosal Dermatitis, Diarrhea, and Dementia). Patients may be hyperpigmented.

Vitamin C (ascorbic acid) deficiency causes scurvy. Ascorbic acid is a vital vitamin in connective tissue formation. Scurvy usually occurs in poverty stricken urban areas. First symptoms are petechial hemorrhages and ecchymoses; then the patient gets hyperkeratotic papules around hair follicles, Sjögren syndrome, hemorrhage into muscles and joints, purpura, and splinter hemorrhages in the nail beds. In children, it affects bone formation and can cause intracerebral hemorrhage. Symptoms improve only when the normal pool is replenished (1.5 - 3 grams).

Vitamin A deficiency is a major cause of blindness in developing countries; night blindness is the earliest symptom of deficiency.

Vitamin D deficiency causes rickets in children and osteomalacia in adults. Decreased vitamin D causes decreased absorption of calcium from the gut and decreased calcium resorption from the kidney. Deficiency also stimulates the release of PTH. Early in the course of the disease, the hypocalcemia is blunted by the increase in PTH which increases absorption from the gut and also leaches calcium from the bones; so even though there is a normal or slightly low serum calcium, the patient still gets the bone problems!

Vitamin E is an antioxidant. Deficiency is usually seen when there is fat malabsorption and also a deficiency of the other fat soluble vitamins. Deficient patients can have areflexia and decreased vibration and position sense which is caused by deterioration of the posterior columns of the spinal cord. Intense research is underway assessing the antioxidant effects of vitamin E on atherosclerotic lesions.

VITAMIN OVERDOSE

Hypervitaminosis A can be caused by eating polar bear liver but more commonly it is a result of over-ingestion of vitamin supplements causing headache and flaky skin. A single massive dose causes abdominal pain, sluggishness, papilledema, and a bulging fontanel in infants. This is followed in a few days with desquamation of the skin and recovery. Chronic over-ingestion (25,000 U/day) is associated with arthralgias, anorexia, dry skin, hair loss, low grade fever, and hepatosplenomegaly.

Vitamin B6 excess can cause a peripheral neuropathy with normal motor and sensory function but absent position and vibration sense.

Hypervitaminosis D results in increased calcium absorption from the bowel, hypercalcemia, and hypercalciuria. It probably increases the tendency for calcium renal stones. The hypercalcemia and hypercalciuria seen in chronic granulomatous diseases (such as sarcoidosis and lymphomas) are due to an equivalent hypervitaminosis D state in which there is increased $1,25 (OH)_2 D$.

Vitamin E is relatively nontoxic. The main trouble with vitamin E is that large doses can cause a marked potentiation of oral anticoagulants.

Vitamin C megadoses increase the possibility of oxalate renal stones and can interfere with the absorption of B12.

High doses of niacin can cause acanthosis nigricans and cholestatic jaundice. The flushing and pruritus often occurring at the start of treatment is prevented by taking aspirin 30 minutes before the niacin.

If the choice is between enteric feeding and TPN, enteric feeding is the better option. The glutamine and short-chained fatty acid substrates (fatty acids are manufactured in the small intestine) in the enteric feedings help maintain the integrity of the small intestinal wall—the loss of which is associated with the onset of multisystem failure. Glutamine is too unstable to be used in TPN. Percutaneous endoscopic gastrostomy is often used in patients who cannot swallow. It is a better alternative to the NG tube and general anesthesia is not required. Contraindications to percutaneous endoscopic gastrostomy are delayed gastric emptying and gastric outlet obstruction. In these cases various types of jejunostomy tubes can be used.

Simple clues to malnutrition:
- Weight/ideal weight < 70%
- Lymphocyte count < 1000/mm^3
- Low albumin
- Low triceps skin fold thickness
- Low urine creatinine to height ratio = (24hr urine excretion of creatinine in μg) ÷ (height in centimeters) < 10 in men, < 6 in women.

Greater than 10% weight loss over 6 months indicates a possibility of malnutrition. Albumin is an indicator of nutritional status but it may also be lower after major trauma or during an infection (due to vascular leakage of albumin or decreased albumin production by the liver). Malnourished patients are typically anergic. Triceps skin fold measurement is good only for long term assessment of nutritional status. Short

notes

term changes may not be meaningful because of changes in hydration and edema.

Indirect calorimetry units that measure oxygen consumption and CO_2 production are more precise and usually better for determining needed calories for in-hospital, critically ill patients.

These questions are to assist you in integrating the information you have just reviewed in this section. These are purposely NOT board-style questions as they are meant to cover a lot of material in minimal space. MedStudy does have board-style Q&As in books and CD-ROM format.

TRUE/FALSE

1) ERCP:
  A. High amylase after ERCP is usually an indication of acute pancreatitis caused by the procedure.
  B. ERCP is indicated in the workup of acute pancreatitis.

  [F, F(only if there are impacted gallstones or lack of clinical improvement in non-alcoholic acute pancreatitis). Note: for these T/F questions, follow along in the book section for clarification]

2) Esophagus:
  A. Achalasia results in decreased tonus of the esophagus and lower esophageal sphincter.
  B. In achalasia, the UGI shows a narrowing at the LES.
  C. Diffuse esophageal spasm is often precipitated by cold or carbonated liquids.
  D. Nutcracker esophagus often causes severe chest pain.
  E. Severity of symptoms correlates with tissue damage in esophagitis.
  F. Barrett esophagus is associated with squamous cell cancer.

  [A=F, B=T, C=T, D=T, E=F, F=F(adenocarcinoma)]

3) Stomach:
  A. Type A gastritis is the most common form of gastritis.
  B. Gastric cancer is usually an adenocarcinoma.
  C. The G-cells make gastric acid.

  [A=F(type B is most common-80%), B=T, C=F(G cells make gastrin which stimulates the parietal cells to make gastric acid.)]

4) PUD:
  A. Smoking decreases healing rate and increases recurrences of both types of PUD.
  B. Smoking does not increase the rate of perforation in PUD.
  C. *H. pylori* is the cause of virtually all gastric ulcers.
  D. In the workup of patients with a gastric ulcer, all should have endoscopy with at least 6 biopsy samples of the ulcer.
  E. With secretin stimulation, ZE patients have a paradoxical decrease in gastrin level.

  [A=T, B=F, C=F(most *duodenal* ulcers), D=F(this is only done with *nonhealing* gastric ulcers), E=F(paradoxical *increase* in gastrin level)]

5) Inflammatory bowel disease:
  A. Toxic megacolon is a complication of ulcerative colitis but not Crohn disease.
  B. Both prednisone and sulfasalazine are okay to give to pregnant patients.
  C. Only azathioprine decreases the relapse rate in Crohn disease.
  D. IBD is more common than colon cancer.
  E. IBD is the most common cause of bloody diarrhea.
  F. There is an increased risk of colon cancer in both UC and Crohn disease.
  G. Surgery is the cure for Crohn disease.
  H. Ulcerative proctitis is identical to early UC but it has no increased risk of cancer.

  [A=F(both UC and Crohn d.), B=T, C=F(aza *and* 6-mercap), D=F, E=F, F=T, G=F(colectomy cures UC but not Crohn disease, H=T]

6) Diarrhea:
  A. A 24-hour fast will stop all osmotic diarrhea except possibly that from surreptitious ingestion of Mg-containing antacids. It will also stop secretory diarrhea due to fatty acids and fat malabsorption.
  B. If a patient with pseudomembranous colitis has a relapse soon after initial treatment, new therapy with a different class of antibiotic should be started.
  C. 3 day quantitative fecal fat is the best screen for malabsorption.
  D. Steatorrhea is defined as > 14 gm/d of fecal fat.
  E. A low xylose test is caused only by small bowel disease.
  F. Celiac sprue is caused by gluten sensitivity and may lead to intestinal lymphoma.
  G. The small bowel biopsy findings in Celiac sprue can be mimicked by acute gastroenteritis.
  H. Some of the abdominal symptoms in Whipple disease are caused by lymphatic obstruction.

  [A=T, B=F(recurrence of the diarrhea is usually due to spores becoming active—so just repeat the same treatment), C=F(Sudan stain of the stool is the best screen for malabsorption, steatorrhea is the best indicator of malabsorption, and the 3 day quantitative test is the gold standard for diagnosis), D=T, E=F(many causes—see text), F=T, G=T, H=T]

7) GI Cancer:
  A. Small (< 2 cm) pedunculated adenomas are more likely to be malignant than large (> 2 cm) sessile ones.
  B. Hyperplastic polyps have only a little malignant potential.
  C. CEA levels are good for checking for intestinal cancer recurrences only if they were elevated before the surgery and decreased after the surgery.
  D. Surgery is the treatment of choice for all forms of intestinal cancer.

  [A=F, B= F(no malignant potential), C= T, D= T]

8) Pancreatitis:
   A. High lipid level may cause a spuriously low amylase level in acute pancreatitis.
   B. A pancreatic pseudocyst should be drained immediately.
   C. A plain film of the abdomen is useless in diagnosing chronic pancreatitis.
   D In diabetes due to chronic pancreatitis, the patient is less susceptible to hypoglycemia.

   [A=T, B= F(surgical drainage is usually indicated if the pseudocyst persists > 1 month), C= F(if a plain film of the abdomen shows calcification of the pancreas, the diagnosis of chronic pancreatitis is made.), D=F(much more susceptible)]

9) Hepatobiliary system:
   A. Cholelithiasis can be caused by hypercholesterolemia.
   B. Primary biliary cirrhosis usually occurs in middle-aged women and about 35% of affected patients are antimitochondrial antibody positive.
   C. Hepatic copper levels are elevated in PBC, Primary sclerosing cholangitis, and Wilson disease.
   D. Primary sclerosing cholangitis is more commonly seen in Crohn disease than in UC.

   [A=F, B= F(90%), C=T, D=F(PSC is strongly associated with colitis—so it is more often seen in UC)]

10) Hepatitis:
   A. Hepatitis B and C are transmitted by blood while A and E are transmitted by the fecal-oral route.
   B. Immune globulin (IG) is recommended for prophylaxis against hepatitis B and A.
   C. Hepatitis B is the only RNA hepatitis virus.
   D. Hepatitis C causes 90% of transfusion associated hepatitis.
   E. Hepatoma is associated with hepatitis B but not C.
   F. Alpha-interferon is the indicated treatment for auto-immune CAH.

   [A=T, B=F(IG for HAV, HBIG for HBV), C=F(HBV is the only DNA hepatitis virus), D=F(not since pre-1990's), E=F(hepatoma is associated with both HBV and HCV), F=F(Alpha interferon is contraindicated in autoimmune CAH—it is indicated in the treatment of Hep B and C CAH)]

11) Cirrhosis:
   A Not more than 1 liter/day should be removed by paracentesis.
   B. Alkalosis and hypokalemia are two precipitating factors for hepatic encephalopathy.

   [A=F(not more than one l/d should be diuresed off), B=T]

12) Hereditary liver disease:
   A. Rotor syndrome is a type of Dubin-Johnson syndrome.
   B. 99% of hemochromatosis patients have cardiac involvement.

   [A=T, B=F(15%)]

---

13) A. Schatzki Ring
    B. Diffuse esophageal spasm
    C. Carcinoma
    D. Scleroderma
    E. Peptic stricture
    F. Achalasia

1. 30 year-old with chest pain and intermittent dysphagia to solids and liquids.
2. 25 year-old with intermittent dysphagia to solids only.
3. Progressive dysphagia to solids and liquids, nocturnal aspiration.
4. Progressive dysphagia to solids only and a history of heartburn.
5. Progressive dysphagia to solids and liquids and a history of heartburn.
6. 75 year-old with progressive dysphagia to solids only.

   [1(B) 2(A-this often has intermittent sx initially) 3(F) 4(E) 5 (D) 6(C)]

14) A. Familial colonic polyposis
    B. Gardner syndrome
    C. Peutz-Jeghers syndrome
    D. Juvenile polyposis

1. No malignant potential
2. 100% risk of cancer.
3. Hamartomas
4. Adenomas

   [1(D) 2(A,B) 3(C,D) 4(A,B)]

15) A. Hydrocortisone enemas
    B. Prednisone
    C. Sulfasalazine
    D. Metronidazole
    E. 6-mercaptopurine
    F. Azathioprine

1. Treatment of choice for mild UC.
2. Decreases relapse rate in Crohn disease.
3. Not effective in mild to moderate UC.
4. Treatment of choice for moderate UC.
5. Steroid sparing.
6. Causes reversible infertility in men.
7. Decreases relapse rate in UC.
8. Safe in pregnancy

   [1(A,C; also mesalamine) 2(E,F) 3(D) 4(B—but not given long-term) 5(E,F) 6(C) 7(A,B,C,E,F; also mesalamine) 8(A,B,C)]

16) A. Gilbert syndrome
    B. Dubin-Johnson syndrome
    C. Crigler-Najjar syndrome
    D. Rotor syndrome
    E. Benign postoperative cholestasis

1. Conjugated hyperbilirubinemia.
2. Unconjugated hyperbilirubinemia.
3. Occurs in 7% of the population.
4. Coarse pigment accumulation in the centrilobular hepato-cytes.
5. Increased unconjugated bilirubin after surgery.
6. Increased conjugated bilirubin after surgery.

[1(B,E,D) 2(A,C) 3(A) 4(B) 5(A) 6(E)]

17) A. Wilson disease
    B. Hemochromatosis
    C. Alpha-1 antitrypsin

1. Always hereditary.
2. Liver transplant is curative.
3. Low serum ceruloplasmin.
4. Early treatment results in a normal lifespan.
5. May be caused by sideroblastic anemia or thalassemia.
6. Psychiatric dysfunction in adolescents.
7. Eye findings are pathognomonic.

[1(A,C) 2(A,C—but note that a patient with Wilson disease can be maintained indefinitely on penicillamine or trientine) 3(A) 4(B) 5(B) 6(A) 7(A)]

18) A. Hepatitis A
    B. Hepatitis B
    C. Hepatitis C
    D. Hepatitis D
    E. Hepatitis E

1. High risk of fulminant hepatitis in third trimester of pregnancy.
2. Requires coexistent hepatitis B to be pathogenic.
3. Caused 90% of transfusion-related hepatitis prior to 1990.
4. No carrier/chronic states.
5. When concurrent with hepatitis B, is often fatal.
6. When acquired as a superinfection in a person with chronic hepatitis B, infection is often severe.
7. 5-7% go on to a chronic carrier state.
8. 60-75% go on to a chronic carrier state.

[1(E) 2(D) 3(C) 4(A,E) 5(C) 6(D) 7(B) 8(C)]

19) A. Zollinger-Ellison (gastrinoma)
    B. G-cell hyperplasia
    C. Post-antrectomy for G-cell hyperplasia
    D. Normal

1. No change in gastrin levels after secretin stimulation.
2. Decreased gastrin in response to secretin stimulation.
3. Increased gastrin in response to secretin stimulation.
4. No change in gastrin level after a protein meal.

[1(C) 2(D - this will also occur if there is retained antrum after antrectomy) 3(A) 4(A)]

20) A. Ulcerative Colitis
    B. Crohn disease
    C. Both
    D. Neither

1. Patchy, transmural, deep ulcers.
2. Always starts in the rectum and spreads up.
3. String sign.
4. Cured surgically.
5. If skin lesions are present, they correlate with disease activity.
6. Associated with intestinal cancer.

[1(B) 2(A) 3(B) 4(A) 5(C) 6(C)]

21) A. Osmotic diarrhea
    B. Secretory diarrhea
    C. Both
    D. Neither

1. isotonic
2. $2[Na+ + K+]$ - serum osmolality > 50
3. Bacterial enterotoxins
4. Celiac disease
5. Antibiotic-associated diarrhea

[1(C) 2(A—osmotic gap > 50 = osmotic, osmotic gap < 50 = secretory) 3(B) 4(C) 5(D)]

22) A. Primary biliary cirrhosis
    B. Primary sclerosing cholangitis
    C. Both
    D. Neither

1. Usually occurs in middle aged women
2. Strong association with colitis
3. Elevated hepatic copper level
4. Antimitochondrial antibody positive
5. Anti-smooth muscle antibody positive
6. High bilirubin and alkaline phosphatase

[1(A) 2(B) 3(C - also Wilson disease) 4(A -90%; occasionally positive in both autoimmune and drug-induced CAH) 5(D - this is positive only in autoimmune CAH) 6(C)]

23) A. B1 deficiency

B. B2 deficiency
C. B6 deficiency
D. B12 deficiency
E. Niacin deficiency
F. Vitamin C deficiency
G. Vitamin A deficiency
H. Vitamin D deficiency
I. Vitamin E deficiency

1. Major cause of blindness
2. Wernicke-Korsakoff
3. Carcinoid syndrome
4. Phenothiazines and tricyclic antidepressants
5. Hemorrhages into joints; splinter hemorrhages; petechiae
6. INH
7. Areflexia; posterior column deterioration
8. Osteomalacia
9. Glossitis, stomatitis, diarrhea, dementia.
10. Glossitis, seizures.
11. Heart failure

[1(G) 2(A) 3(E) 4(B) 5(F) 6(C,E) 7(I) 8(H) 9(E) 10(C) 11(A)]

SHORT CASE SCENARIOS

24) A 40 year-old presents with a 3 month history of dyspepsia relieved by eating. No other symptoms. What workup is indicated?

[None; workup only if the symptoms persist on antacids AND if the ALARM signals are absent (see text)]

25) Patient has a long history of dyspepsia and now has difficulty swallowing solids. What test should be performed now?

[EGD to check for probable peptic stricture.]

26) Teenager with acne presents with dyspepsia and dysphagia. What is the probable diagnosis? What is the workup? What is the treatment?

[Doxycycline-induced esophagitis; none; symptomatic treatment and stop the doxycycline.]

27) 70 year-old drinker with a history of progressive dysphagia—initially to solids and now to liquids. What is the initial test in the workup and what is the most likely diagnosis?

[EGD; cancer is most likely cause. Consider this in anybody over 65—especially if they are drinkers or smokers.]

28) 50 year-old with recent onset of epigastric burning pain. Normal CBC. Normal stomach acidity. Normal EKG. EGD found only gastritis. Is this more likely type A or type B gastritis? Is it likely to be associated with *H. pylori*?

[Type B; yes]

29) A patient with Crohn disease is 3 months post-surgery during which 15 inches of his distal ileum was removed. He develops diarrhea. What is the probable cause? How is it treated?

[This patient probably has bile acid-induced diarrhea which is treated with bile acid sequestrants such as cholestyramine. When (roughly) more than 100 cm of distal ileum is removed, steatorrhea results and a low fat diet is started. Infrequently, medium-chain triglycerides are also used.]

30) A patient presents with a history of intermittent frequent loose stools for years. His stool has fecal WBCs and blood. C+S and O+P are negative on 3 stool specimens. On colonoscopy, mucosal inflammation from the rectum to the proximal sigmoid colon is found. What is the diagnosis? What is the initial treatment? What is used if the initial treatment doesn't work? Is this patient at risk for cancer?

[U.C.; Oral sulfasalazine, oral or rectal mesalamine, or hydrocortisone enemas; Prednisone; Yes—colon cancer.]

31) 50 year-old patient has a 3 year history of chronic pancreatitis caused by ETOH. She had onset of smelly diarrhea 2 months ago. 3 day quantitative fecal fat was 60 grams. What is the probable cause of the diarrhea. What tests can be used to confirm this diagnosis?

[Pancreatic insufficiency; xylose absorption test, qualitative stool exam revealing undigested muscle fibers, neural fat, and split fat. The undigested muscle fibers indicates impaired digestion. It is further confirmed by a positive response to treatment with pancreatic enzymes.]

32) 50 year-old patient presents with 1 day history of fever, left lower quadrant abdominal pain, and bloody stools. She has rebound tenderness in the area of pain. Which one of the following are true?

A. A sigmoid mass may be found on physical exam.
B. The most likely diagnosis is the most common cause of GI bleeding in the elderly.
C. The probable problem may cause colonic bowel obstruction.
D. If not done previously, workup for colon cancer is required after symptoms resolve.
E. All of the above

[E]

33) A 45 year-old woman presents with complaints of fever and malaise for 2 weeks and jaundice for 1 week. She lives in a poor socioeconomic area. She says she last did IV drugs "a year ago." Blood tests show: ALT 1300, AST 1250, Bilirubin 4.5, Anti-HAV IgG positive, Anti-HAV IgM negative, HBsAg neg, HBeAg neg, HBcAg neg, Anti-HBsAg neg. Which of the following are true? More than one answer may be correct.

A. The patient has hepatitis A.
B. The patient does not have hepatitis B.
C. Hepatitis C is the most probable cause.
D. Primary biliary cirrhosis is the most probable cause.
E. None of the above

[E. The patient does not have hepatitis A (else the Anti-HAV IgM would be positive). The patient may be in the "window" for hepatitis B studies; an anti-HBc IgM should be done. Primary biliary cirrhosis may present with a high bilirubin but the liver transaminases are not this elevated. Assuming that the patient is exaggerating the time since her last IV street drugs, hepatitis B is more likely than C. HIV testing should also be done.]

OPEN-ENDED QUESTIONS

34) What are 3 tests which may be used in the workup of GE reflux?

[If the patient is resistant to initial treatment or if there are alarm signals, then perform endoscopy. If the EGD is normal and the patient has refractory symptoms, then perform either 24 hour intraesophageal pH monitor or a Bernstein test]

35) What is the most common connective tissue disease affecting the esophagus?

[Scleroderma.]

36) Should a patient with pernicious anemia have periodic endoscopic exams?

[No. Because the incidence of gastric cancer is so low, the 3XN increase in gastric cancer is not enough to warrant periodic endoscopic exams.]

37) Carcinoids often cause intolerance to what chemical?

[ETOH]

38) With what 4 hypergastrinemic states is gastric carcinoid associated?

[Pernicious anemia, chronic gastritis, ZE, renal failure, hyperthyroidism, and vitiligo.]

39) Name the neurocrine, endocrine, and paracrine stimuli for gastric acid production.

[Neurocrine: vagus nerve; endocrine: gastrin; and paracrine: histamine.]

40) Which medication is preferred in patients with severe renal disease sucralfate, H2 blockers, or proton pump inhibitors?

[Of the drugs listed, sucralfate is preferred because it also binds PO4.]

41) What are the primary treatments for *H. pylori* infection?

[Usually triple drug therapy is used—two antibiotics and a proton pump inhibitor. A good one with an eradication rate of about 90% is O-CLAM (omeprazole 20mg + clarithromycin 500mg + amoxicillin 1g—bid x 10d).]

42) Which is better (and why) for diagnosing cause of an UGI bleed—UGI or endoscopy?

[Endoscopy. This will find Mallory-Weiss tear, stress gastritis, and Osler-Weber-Rendu syndrome which the UGI usually misses.]

43) If a patient with a gastric ulcer also has achlorhydria after the stimulus of a meal, is the ulcer more likely to be malignant?

[Yes.]

44) What is Stress Related Mucosal Damage and what 2 classes of drugs are used to treat it?

[SRMD is PUD or gastritis associated with critical illness. Both antacids and H2-receptor antagonists are effective treatments.]

45) Which extraintestinal manifestations of IBD do not improve with improvement of the colitis?

[Primary sclerosing cholangitis, uveitis, and ankylosing spondylitis.]

46) What are the prednisone-sparing drugs used in IBD?

[6-mercaptopurine and azathioprine.]

47) What are two important side effects of sulfasalazine?

[Leukopenia and reversible infertility in men.]

48) Which drugs decrease the relapse rate in Crohn disease? Which in UC?

[The only drugs that decrease the relapse rate in Crohn disease are azathioprine and 6-mercaptopurine, while ALL of the standard drugs decrease the relapse rate in UC!]

49) What is the "string sign"?

[In Crohn disease, the terminal ileum can become so edematous that the lumen is compressed and shows up as a string of contrast. The edema pushes the rest of the bowel away so the "string" shows up well.]

50) Which inflammatory bowel disease is most likely to cause bile acid-induced diarrhea?

[Crohn disease (not UC) has problems related to disease/resection of the terminal ileum such as oxalate kidney stones, cholesterol gallstones, B12 deficiency, hypocalcemia (vitamin D malabsorption), bile acid induced diarrhea (< 100 cm ileum removed), and low bile acid diarrhea (> 100 cm ileum removed).]

51) When is colectomy recommended for UC?

[Colectomy for UC is reserved for: 1) fulminant UC not responsive to steroids or antibiotics and 2) if the patient has dysplasia in a mass lesion or high-grade dysplasia in flat mucosa.]

52) What is the difference between antibiotic-associated diarrhea and antibiotic-associated colitis?

[Antibiotic associated diarrhea is a dysmotility problem; whereas, antibiotic associated colitis is pseudomembranous colitis caused by *Clostridium difficile*.]

53) In invasive diarrhea: Which is the most common type? Which causes joint aches? Which is seen in patients with sickle cell disease or with achlorhydria?

[Most common invasive diarrhea is caused by Campylobacter. Yersinia is associated with joint pains and rash. Salmonella is seen in patients with sickle cell disease or achlorhydria.]

54) Why are bronchial carcinoids more symptomatic than ones in other sites?

[Bronchial carcinoids dump vasoactive mediators directly into the arterial circulation causing more symptoms (flushing, hypotension, tachycardia, and explosive diarrhea.]

55) What is the usual cause of diarrhea in an AIDS patient with weight loss and diarrhea but without fever? What are the other possible causes? With fever?

[If the AIDS patient has diarrhea and weight loss without fever, suspect *Cryptosporidia* (usual cause), *E. histolytica*, *Giardia*, *Isospora*, *Strongyloides*, and HIV enteropathy. Note that all these organisms are noninvasive. With fever, think of *Mycobacterium*, *Campylobacter*, *Salmonella*, *Cryptococcus*, *Histoplasma*, and CMV.]

56) What are the two main etiologies of malabsorption and how do you differentiate them?

[Malabsorption is either caused by decreased mucosal transport or by decreased digestion due to pancreatic insufficiency. They are differentiated by the xylose absorption test. Know this test!!]

57) If a patient has 100 gm/d of fecal fat, the diagnosis is _____. Will the xylose absorption test be normal or abnormal?

[Pancreatic insufficiency. Xylose absorption is not dependent on breakdown by pancreatic enzymes so the xylose absorption test in normal in pancreatic insufficiency.]

58) Which other substances are absorbed similarly to d-xylose?

[The absorption of carotene, vitamin K, vitamin D, folate, and iron are also, like xylose, independent of pancreatic enzyme digestion.]

59) If you see a small bowel biopsy with foamy macrophages, what disease comes to mind?

[Whipple disease.]

60) At what age are the screening exams for colon cancer started? What screening exams are recommended and how often?

[Current screening recommendations are to do yearly rectal exam and stool guaiacs, and every 3 year flexible sigmoidoscopies after age 50. Start at age 40 if there is moderately increased risk (i.e., positive family history). With high risk patients, use colonoscopy only; this is the best method for detecting colon cancer.]

61) What is the most common cause of small bowel obstruction? Of colonic obstruction?

[The most frequent cause of small intestine obstruction is adhesions. In decreasing order, the most common causes of colonic obstruction are: carcinoma…then diverticulitis… then volvulus.]

62) What is the most common form of intestinal ischemia?

[Ischemic colitis. Especially consider this in patients with CHF. Thumbprinting is seen on x-ray or BE.]

63) What physical exam technique allows you to differentiate between neurogenic and acquired megacolon?

[The digital rectal exam. In megacolon due to psychogenic constipation, the digital exam reveals a rectum distended with stool. In aganglionic megacolon the rectal vault is empty!]

64) What is the usual course of a pancreatic mass in a patient with pancreatitis?

[A pancreatic mass in a patient with acute pancreatitis usually resolves—but it could also be a pancreatic pseudocyst which, if it persists > 1 month, will probably require surgical drainage. Associated fever and shock suggests an abscess.]

65) What are the most common causes of acute pancreatitis? Of chronic pancreatitis?

[Acute pancreatitis: alcohol abuse and gallstones. Chronic pancreatitis: chronic ETOH ingestion.]

66) Besides pancreatitis, name 6 other causes of abdominal pain associated with an elevated amylase.

[Acute pancreatitis, acute cholecystitis, intestinal infarction, diabetic ketoacidosis, perforated ulcer, salpingitis, and ectopic pregnancy! Other causes of hyperamylasemia are increased salivary amylase and macroamylasemia (a benign condition due to a low urinary excretion of amylase).]

67) How should diabetes due to chronic pancreatitis be controlled—tight or loose? Why?

[Loose. These patients are very prone to hypoglycemia because they no longer produce glucagon.]

68) What is the proper treatment for a patient with gallstones but no history of symptoms?

[No treatment is indicated.]

69) When is the HIDA scan used?

[The HIDA scan is best used for confirming acute cystic duct obstruction (i.e., acute cholecystitis).]

70) In which diseases is anti-smooth muscle antibody usually found and in which is the antimitochondrial antibody usually found?

[Antimitochondrial antibody is seen in 90% of primary biliary cirrhosis patients. It is occasionally seen in chronic active hepatitis of both the drug-induced and autoimmune types. Anti-smooth muscle antibody is seen only in autoimmune CAH.]

71) Name 3 diseases with an elevated hepatic copper level.

[Primary sclerosing cholangitis, Wilson disease, and primary biliary cirrhosis.]

72) Primary sclerosing cholangitis has a strong association with what disease?

[Colitis—either ulcerative colitis or Crohn disease involving the colon.]

73) In what two diseases is fatty liver microvesicular?

[The fat globules are microvesicular in acute fatty liver of pregnancy and in Reye syndrome. All other types of fatty liver—from ETOH, protein malnutrition, AODM, obesity, or prolonged IV hyperalimentation—store fat in large cytoplasmic fat globules (i.e., macrovesicular).]

74) Which hepatitis viruses are spread by fecal-oral route? By blood?

[Fecal-oral: hepatitis A and E. Blood transmitted: hepatitis B,C, and D.]

75) Is the hepatitis D virus infection less severe if acquired by a hepatitis B carrier (vs. acute HBV infection)?

[Hepatitis D usually will not make an acute HBV infection much worse but, if acquired as a superinfection in a HBV carrier, the infection is frequently very severe.]

76) Name the "ABCDE" causes of chronic hepatitis.

[A: autoimmune; B: hepatitis B; C: hepatitis C; D: drugs; E: et cetera, which includes alcohol, alpha-1 antitrypsin deficiency, Wilson disease, and hemochromatosis.]

77) What is the treatment for chronic hepatitis B? For chronic hepatitis C?

[Alpha interferon is the only medical treatment for the chronic active forms of hepatitis B and hepatitis C.]

78) What is a serologic marker for hepatoma?

[Alpha-fetoprotein.]

79) What is the treatment for esophageal variceal hemorrhage? What is given to decrease rebleed?

[Primary therapy for active variceal bleed is endoscopic sclerotherapy. Vasopressin with nitroglycerin is used if endoscopy is not available. TIPSS (transjugular intrahepatic portal systemic shunt) in indicated if the patient rebleeds. Propranolol is prophylactic.]

80) In ascites, what does an elevated serum-to-ascites albumin gradient (> 1.1) indicate? In what types of ascites is there high ascitic fluid protein level?

[Portal hypertension is indicated by a serum-to-ascites albumin gradient >1.1 (i.e., low ascites albumin level) and is seen in ascites due to RHF, cirrhosis, fulminant liver failure, Budd-Chiari syndrome, and myxedema. An elevated ascites protein level (> 2.5) is seen in cardiac ascites, nephrotic syndrome, pancreatitis, tuberculosis peritonitis, and peritoneal carcinomatosis. With all except the first, the SAAG is < 1.1—(i.e., high ascites protein level).]

81) Name 5 factors that may precipitate hepatic encephalopathy. Does NH_3 or NH_4^+ precipitate it? Why?

[Hepatic encephalopathy may be precipitated by GI bleed, pneumonia, increased dietary protein, low potassium, sedatives, and also alkalosis which increases ammonia/ammonium ratio (NH_3/NH_4^+). Only the non-ionized form—NH_3 (ammonia)—crosses the blood-brain barrier.]

82) If an alcoholic presents with bleeding and an increased PT, and if it is easily correctable by vitamin K, is the cause liver disease?

[No—the cause is malabsorption.]

83) Why is only conjugated bilirubin passed in the urine?

[Conjugated bilirubin is less tightly bound to albumin than unconjugated bilirubin. The 5% unbound portion of conjugated bilirubin easily passes into the urine. So—bilirubinuria means conjugated hyperbilirubinemia. Because bilirubin is conjugated in the liver, bilirubinuria is an indication of cholestasis.]

84) If a patient has a postop increase in conjugated bilirubin, what is the probable cause? If the increase is in unconjugated bilirubin, what is the probable cause?

[Increased conjugated bilirubin after a major surgery indicates benign post-operative cholestasis. Increased unconjugated bilirubin after major surgery indicates Gilbert syndrome.]

85) What blood tests suggest hemochromatosis? What test confirms it? How is it treated? Will treatment improve cardiac function?

[Diagnosis of hemochromatosis is suggested by high serum Fe, ferritin, and transferrin levels. Only a liver biopsy confirms the diagnosis. Treatment of hemochromatosis results in decreased skin pigmentation, improved cardiac function, and prolonged life expectancy. If already lost, secondary sex characteristics will not return (the damage is done! Treatment is periodic phlebotomies).

MedStudy

The Internal Medicine Review

Infectious Disease

Authored by Robert A. Hannaman, MD

Many thanks to

Alan A. Morganstein, MD
Glendale, California

and

J. Thomas Cross, Jr., MD, MPH
Associate Director of Education
MedStudy
Colorado Springs, Colorado

Infectious Disease Advisors

Note: The Table of Contents for this section is located in front of the book.

CYTOKINES

Cytokines are produced by lymphocytes (which produce lymphokines), neutrophils, monocytes (monokines), and macrophages.

Interleukin-1 (IL-1) is a lymphokine which was historically known as "endogenous pyrogen" and mediates the generation of fever in the hypothalamus. IL-1 stimulates neutrophils to reproduce and congregate (chemotaxis), T-cells to produce other lymphokines, and B-cells to produce antibodies, and it causes fever! Interleukin-1 also causes T-cells to produce interleukin-2 which, in turn, stimulates the production of all the T-cell types (helpers, suppressors, and killers).

Interferons: Another class of cytokines, the interferons, have three types: alpha, beta, and gamma. The most potent interferon in the immune system is gamma, which is produced by T-cells (both helper and suppressor). Gamma interferon both decreases virus-infected cell proliferation and activates macrophages. Some macrophages also produce interferon. (Again: macrophages and T-cells produce interferon.)

Growth factor is the newer name which covers the interleukins, colony-stimulating factors, and erythropoietin. It has been found that these substances are the actual molecules which combine with the cell surface receptors and stimulate the cells. More in Hematology.

Unregulated cytokine activation is felt to be the origin of SIRS (systemic inflammatory response syndrome). SIRS may have an infectious or noninfectious etiology. When infection is suspected/shown, the condition is called sepsis. Tumor necrosis factor (TNF) may be the most important mediator. TNF is a cytokine released by neutrophils, monocytes, and macrophages in response to endotoxin (lipopolysaccharide; LPS). Once released, TNF amplifies the signal LPS and transmits it to other cells.

Drotrecogin alpha (activated) (Xigris®) is a new antithrombotic agent (recombinant form of activated protein C) that improves survival in patients with severe sepsis—i.e., Apache II scores ≥ 25.

NEUTROPENIA

Neutropenia (granulocytopenia) occurs in leukemia, bone marrow transplant, ablative chemotherapy, metastases to the bone marrow, and overwhelming sepsis. Previously, the most common infections in patients with neutropenia were gram-negative but this has shifted to gram-positive organisms—probably due to the widespread use of third-generation cephalosporins and due to increased central venous catheter use. Especially consider *S. aureus*. Gram-negative infections are still common. *Corynebacterium jeikeium* (JK) and fungi (*Candida*, *Aspergillus*, and *Mucor*) also may occur. The tendency for infection is directly proportional to the amount of granulocytopenia less than 500! If the patient is not neutropenic, but has a history of recurrent staphylococcal skin infections, recurrent lung infections, and lymphadenitis, suspect a granulocyte dysfunction.

If a neutropenic patient presents with fever, you must initially cover for gram-negative organisms. Some say also always cover for staph because skin and oral organisms also are causes of infection. If there is the slightest suspicion of staph, cover for it. Antibiotics of choice in a neutropenic person with fever are:

• Aminoglycoside with a beta-lactam; usually an antipseudomonal PCN (ticarcillin-clavulanate, piperacillin-tazobactam)
• Antipseudomonal cephalosporin: ceftazidime (3rd generation) or cefepime (4th generation), or
• Imipenem-cilastatin
• Also used, and some believe just as good, is a wide-spectrum beta-lactam alone—ceftazidime or IMP/cilastatin. Note that the ceftazidime has no staph coverage.

Vancomycin is not required for initial treatment of neutropenia. If the antibiotics do not appear to be working after 5-7 days, add amphotericin B; if the patient has preexisting renal insufficiency, i.e., creatinine > 3, consider a liposomal amphotericin B instead. Prophylactic antibiotics are not used; although prophylactic quinolones have been shown to decrease the number of serious gram-negative infections, they do not affect survival, so as yet they are not used. Always start antibiotics in a febrile neutropenic patient immediately after blood cultures are drawn.

HUMORAL DEFICIENCIES

Humoral deficiencies (multiple myeloma, asplenia, ALL, CLL, and AIDS) are usually associated with infections caused by encapsulated organisms—especially pneumococcus, meningococcus, and *Haemophilus influenzae*. With acquired hypogammaglobulinemia (common variable immunodeficiency), patients have recurrent sinus and pulmonary infections (often pneumococcus) and recurrent diarrhea (frequently due to *Giardia*). The rule of thumb is if a person has recurrent giardiasis x 3, then check for humoral deficiency. Note that AIDS patients have a humoral deficiency in addition to the T-cell deficiency because the decrease in CD4 cells decreases the normal suppressive effect that CD4 cells have on B cells, and there is an overproduction of nonspecific immunoglobulins—which "gum up the works."

The spleen is intimately involved with humoral immunity. Patients with actual or effective asplenia have the same infections as those with the above humoral deficiencies. Babesiosis and malaria are much more severe in splenectomized patients. This is easy to remember because babesiosis and malaria are similar in other ways—they are both intra-RBC protozoan parasites. Overwhelming *Streptococcus pneumoniae* infection is particularly associated with splenectomy.

IgA blocks viral attachment to mucosal surfaces and IgG blocks viral attachment to host cells. Patients with IgA deficiency often have atopic diseases (asthma, rhinitis...), are more susceptible to giardiasis, and some (those with associated IgG2 deficiency) have increased mucosal infections such as giardiasis, otitis media, pneumonia, and sinusitis—

notes REVIEW ATB CLASSES

the last 3 usually with encapsulated organisms such as *Strep pneumoniae* and *H. influenzae*.

COMPLEMENT DEFICIENCY

Complement—C1, C2, and C4 deficiency cause decreased activation of complement via the classical pathway. Although the alternative pathway takes up some of the slack, these patients still have recurrent sinopulmonary infections (and ear infections when young) caused by encapsulated bacteria. There also is an increased incidence of rheumatoid diseases—especially SLE! C2 deficiency is the most common deficiency in North American whites and should be considered in patients with early-onset SLE.

C3 deficiency results in severe bacterial infections.

C5-C9 deficiency (late complement deficiency) causes infections similar to those in patients with humoral deficiencies or splenectomies—*H. influenzae*, pneumococci and gono- meningococci. Know that patients with late complement deficiency additionally have a unique susceptibility to develop meningococcemia. Because of this, any patient with meningococcemia should be checked for a terminal complement deficiency (about 15% have it—check a CH50 or CH100). The complement cascade is discussed in the Allergy/Immunology section.

T-CELL DEFICIENCY

T-cell deficient patients (AIDS, Hodgkin lymphoma if T-cell derived, T-cell variant of ALL, on steroids or alkylating agents, post organ transplant) are more susceptible to
• Fungi (including *Pneumocystis*)
• *Listeria monocytogenes*
• *Nocardia*
• *Mycobacteria*
• Viruses (especially CMV and Herpes zoster)
• Protozoa (Toxoplasma)
• Helminths (*Strongyloides*)

Transplant patients have decreased cellular immunity due to the required immunosuppressants. *Toxoplasma gondii* infection (pg 2-17) is usually due to a reactivation during immunosuppression. CMV (pg 2-22) is a very common infection 1-4 months after an organ transplant. Note that there is no increased tendency for infection with Staph, Strep, or gram-negative organisms although they still commonly occur.

More on post-transplant infections. As mentioned, these patients have decreased cell-mediated immunity due to immunosuppressive drugs. Certain infections tend to occur in these patients during a fairly specific period of time after the transplant.
• In the first month, the causes of infections are the usual nosocomial postop bacterial infections. One other early infection is Herpes simplex; HSV reactivates in 2/3 of sero-

Table 2-1: Post transplant infections (T cell deficient)	
INFECTIONS IN POST-TRANSPLANT PATIENTS	
Months after transplant	Infectious Organisms
0 to 1	Usual postop nosocomial pneumonias and infections (Gram neg)
1.5	Herpes reactivation
1 to 4	Protozoa (PCP, toxo, strongyloides), fungi, CMV*, Mycobacterium, Listeria, Hepatitis B, Nocardia.
2 to 6	Viruses (Varicella zoster, EBV, Hepatitis C)
4 or more	Cryptococcus neoformans

positive transplant patients within 6 weeks of transplant! Prophylaxis with acyclovir or famciclovir is usually given.
• Between 1-4 months after transplant, look for the infections mentioned above for T-cell immunodeficient patients. Especially consider: TB, *Listeria*, CMV (common), hepatitis B, *Nocardia*, *Toxoplasma*, and *Pneumocystis*.
• From 2-6 months postop, viruses are the major infection. These include varicella-zoster virus, Epstein-Barr virus, and Hepatitis C. *Cryptococcus neoformans* appears from about the 4th month onward. In transplant patients with symptoms of meningitis, include the CSF cryptococcal antigen test and/or India ink test in addition to the other CSF tests. (See Table 2-1)

Question: what previous infections or organisms might reactivate in a person with impaired cellular immunity? Answer: *Nocardia*, TB, *Cryptococcus*, Blastomycosis, Histoplasmosis, Coccidioidomycosis, and *Strongyloides*.

ANTIBIOTIC THERAPY
OVERVIEW

REVIEW OF PROTEIN SYNTHESIS

Most antibiotics work either by interrupting protein synthesis or cell wall synthesis (See Figure 2-1). First let's look at a review of protein synthesis.

Protein Synthesis: Transcription:

The DNA particle must be unwound from its supercoiled arrangement before it can be "read" by RNA polymerase. This involves cutting the strand, holding onto the cut ends to prevent them being damaged, allowing the double helix to uncoil and the DNA to be copied, and then precisely gluing the cut ends back together again. The key enzyme that carries out this process in bacteria is DNA gyrase.

RNA polymerase moves along a section of DNA (a gene), uncoiled by the DNA gyrase and, following the coded messages on the deoxyribonucleotides, forms a string of complemen-

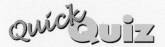

Quick Quiz

1) Which immunodeficiency should you check for in a patient with meningococcemia?

2) What type of infection is most likely to occur within the 1st month of a heart transplant?

3) Which organism would you be concerned about 5 months out from a kidney transplant?

4) What *previous* infections occur in patients with impaired cellular immunity?

tary-paired ribonucleotides, i.e., a piece of RNA—more specifically pre-mRNA. With the removal of an intron the pre-mRNA becomes mRNA (messenger RNA). This is called transcription because the DNA code is transcribed into a complementary RNA code.

Protein Synthesis: Translation:

Ribosomes are the translation units that convert the coded message in the mRNA to a specific sequence of amino acids. A 30S ribosomal subunit attaches to the mRNA at the "ribosome binding site" and then moves along it until it reaches the start codon (AUG). Here a tRNA (with anticodon UAC) carrying an altered methionine (f-Met) binds with this subunit and mRNA to form the "initiation complex". A 50S ribosomal subunit then comes along and binds to this complex to form the 70S ribosome.

Amino acid-specific transfer RNAs (tRNA) attach to the 20 amino acids used in making protein. The bottom loop of these "inverted cloverleaf-shaped" tRNAs have 3 unpaired bases called anticodons.

As the 70S ribosome moves along the mRNA, tRNAs attach

one at a time, bringing these amino acids with them. These amino acids are bound together forming a gradually lengthening protein chain.

When the ribosome reaches the end of the coded message, translation stops. The ribosomal subunits then separate and detach from the mRNA, and the completed protein is released.

ANTIBIOTICS WHICH BLOCK PROTEIN SYNTHESIS

There! Now we can see what is affected by the antibiotics that interfere with protein synthesis:

Rifampin binds to RNA polymerase and blocks initiation of the transcription of DNA to mRNA.

Quinolone antibiotics specifically target the DNA gyrase of bacteria. This allows the DNA gyrase to cut the double helix but then prevents the cut ends from being re-joined.

Metronidazole, a very important anti-anaerobic and anti-protozoal agent, probably has a similar primary mode of action to the quinolones, although it also affects cell membrane function.

Aminoglycosides bind irreversibly (bacteriocidal) to the 30S subunit and prevent the 50S subunit from attaching.

Tetracyclines bind reversibly to the 30S subunit, distorting it so that the anticodons of the tRNAs cannot align properly with the codons on the mRNA.

Oxazolidinones is a new class of antibiotic of which linezolid (Zyvox ™) is the first available. The drug binds to the 50S ribosomal subunit thereby preventing attachment to the initiation complex.

Macrolides bind reversibly to the 50S subunit. They prevent peptide bond formation between the amino acids and hence

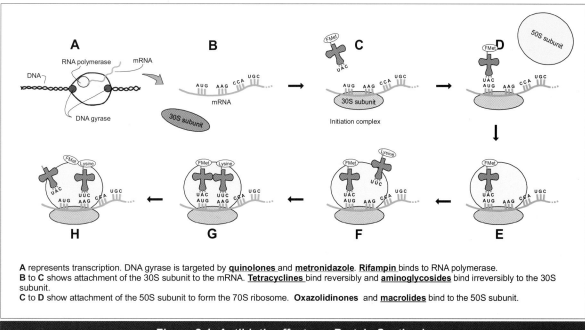

A represents transcription. DNA gyrase is targeted by **quinolones** and **metronidazole**. **Rifampin** binds to RNA polymerase.
B to **C** shows attachment of the 30S subunit to the mRNA. **Tetracyclines** bind reversibly and **aminoglycosides** bind irreversibly to the 30S subunit.
C to **D** show attachment of the 50S subunit to form the 70S ribosome. **Oxazolidinones** and **macrolides** bind to the 50S subunit.

Figure 2-1: Antibiotic effects on Protein Synthesis

notes

keep the 70S ribosome from translocating down the mRNA.

ANTIBIOTICS AFFECTING CELL WALL SYNTHESIS

Peptidoglycan is an exclusively bacterial polymer and is a component of bacterial cell walls. There are a variety of antibiotics that act at one or more stages of peptidoglycan synthesis.

Beta-lactams (see next section) are a class of antibiotics which focuses on attacking the cell wall. They contain a structure similar to that in the amino acids which cross-link and stabilize the bacterium cell wall. Because there is no analogous structure in human cells, these antibiotics can be given at much higher doses without fear of toxicity.

Also:

To replicate DNA, folic acid is required. Bacteria are required to make their own folic acid from paraaminobenzoic acid (PABA). Trimethoprim and the sulfonamides block this process.

Know: Antibacterial agents must be 'cidal for effective treatment of endocarditis, meningitis, and for treatment of infected neutropenic patients. Bactericidal antibiotics are the beta-lactams (PCNs, imipenem, and cephalosporins), fluoroquinolones, vancomycin, aminoglycosides, rifampin, and metronidazole. Bacteriostatic agents are erythromycin, tetracycline, and clindamycin. Chloramphenicol is unusual in that it is normally bacteriostatic but it is 'cidal against *H. influenzae*, pneumococci and meningococci!

BETA-LACTAM ANTIBIOTICS

Overview

The first of the beta-lactam antibiotics was Penicillin (PCN) and now includes the semisynthetic PCNs (methicillin, oxacillin, and cloxacillin), carbapenems, and cephalosporins. Because the bacteria rupture when the integrity of the cell wall is decreased, these drugs are also bactericidal.

Penicillins

Penicillin, as noted above, has the beta-lactam ring. It is very active against meningococci, most streptococci (groups A and B, viridans group, and *S. pneumoniae*) *Pasteurella* (dog and esp. cat bites), *Listeria*, and many *Neisseria* species. It is also active against many anaerobes (such as *Clostridium*), but not *B. fragilis*. Know that even though PCN is indicated for meningococcal infections, rifampin or quinolones are better for eradication of the carrier state. Rifampin concentrates in the upper respiratory mucosa.

PCN is still the drug of choice for many infections:
• periodontal infections
• erysipeloid   • group A and group B strep

• rat-bite fever   • yaws
• leptospirosis   • syphilis
• actinomycosis
• meningococcal meningitis and meningococcemia

Ampicillin has a similar spectrum as PCN, but its spectrum extends to include certain gram-negative rods—especially some *E. coli*, *H. influenzae*, *Salmonella*, *Shigella*, and *Proteus mirabilis*. However, it does not get *Klebsiella* and many of the *H. influenzae*, *E. coli*, and *P. mirabilis* are resistant to it. Ampicillin is the drug of choice for:
• *Listeria monocytogenes* meningitis
• Salmonellosis—if sensitive
• UTIs due to susceptible organisms
• Enterococcal infections

Penicillinase-resistant semisynthetic penicillins like nafcillin and cloxacillin are needed against *S. aureus* because 85% have beta-lactamase (Note: penicillinase is just a specific type of beta-lactamase). Unfortunately there has been a rapidly expanding resistance in staphylococci to these (i.e., "methicillin-resistant"). Nafcillin is similar to methicillin, but it is not as likely to cause interstitial nephritis (so methicillin is rarely used). These (nafcillin and cloxacillin) are drugs of choice only for
• Staphylococcal infections.

Antipseudomonal PCNs (AP-PCN; ticarcillin-clavulanate, piperacillin-tazobactam) are better against the gram-negative organisms (including *Pseudomonas*) and anaerobes (including *B. fragilis*). Like ampicillin—only better. They are the only PCN drugs effective against infections caused by:
• P. aeruginosa   • Acinetobacter

Cephalosporins

Note:

Cephalosporins also contain the beta-lactam ring but are penicillinase resistant. In general, cephalosporins have no activity against enterococci, *Listeria*, and methicillin-resistant staphylococci.

...1st Generation

First-generation cephalosporins (cefazolin, cephalothin, cephapirin) are active against most *Staph* (including the lactamase-producing strains, excluding the methicillin-resistant strains), and most *Strep*. Really no anaerobic activity. First generation also get many of the community acquired *E. coli*, *Klebsiella*, and *Proteus* (the gram-negative coverage is superior to ampicillin). Cephalothin increases the nephrotoxicity of concurrently administered aminoglycosides. Commonly given for:
• Skin and soft tissue infections
• Some surgical prophylaxis

...2nd Generation

All second-generation cephalosporins are more active against the gram-negative organisms (e.g., good against *H. flu*) and less active against gram-positive bacteria.

notes

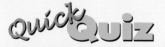

Quick Quiz

1) Oxacillin is the drug of choice for which type of infection?

2) Is a 4th generation cephalosporin useful for an infection due to *Listeria*? What about a 2nd generation?

3) What is given as empiric therapy for suspected bacterial meningitis in a 40 year old? A neonate? The elderly?

4) Write out and memorize the spectrums of the antibiotics.

Parenteral: All of the 2nd generation cephalosporins (Cefoxitin, Cefotetan, Cefamandole, etc. (EXCEPT Cefuroxime-Zinacef®) have variable activity against gut anaerobes. None of the 2nd generation cephalosporins consistently cross into the CSF so are not used to treat meningitis.

These have good activity against *H. influenzae*, *Neisseria*, and gram-positive organisms. They are among drugs of choice for:

• PID
• Abdominal surgery

Know that 3rd generation cephalosporins have largely replaced 2nd generation except for abdominal/pelvic infections because of their anaerobic coverage.

...3rd Generation

Third-generation cephalosporins are especially resistant to beta-lactamase and are especially effective against *N. gonorrhoeae* and *H. influenzae*. They also get most of the *Enterobacteriaceae* (*E. coli*, *Klebsiella*, *Proteus*, *Enterobacter*, and *Serratia*). They are not as active against *S. aureus* as the 1st generation. Of the cephalosporins, only some third-generations are active against *Pseudomonas*—especially ceftazidime (Fortaz®). Ceftriaxone (Rocephin®) has the longest half-life.

There are 4 of the third-generation cephalosporins which can cross an inflamed blood-brain barrier and so are indicated as the primary therapy for meningitis caused by Enterobacteriaceae; these are ceftriaxone, cefotaxime (Claforan®), ceftizoxime (Cefizox®), and ceftazidime.

Remember that ceftriaxone is used as a single agent for empiric treatment of meningitis while lab results are pending (except in neonatal, elderly, and pregnant patients—ampicillin added; and presumed *S. pneumoniae* meningitis—add vancomycin).

There is emerging resistance to third-generation cephalosporins in many bacteria so they are not recommended for routine treatment of community-acquired infections except for community acquired pneumonia (first-line) because they are good against PCN-resistant streptococcal pneumonia.

...4th Generation

"Fourth" generation cephalosporin. Cefepime (Maxipime®) is a broad-spectrum antibiotic with enhanced stability to cephalosporinases. It has the gram-negative activity of third generation cephalosporins and gram-positive activity of first generation cephalosporins. Plus it has good anaerobic coverage! ($1 + 2 + 3 = 4$—it covers all organisms *combined* of the 1st through 3rd generations).

Carbapenems

Imipenem is a carbapenem antibiotic and is a very broad spectrum antibiotic. It is very active against *B. fragilis*. It kills most *Enterobacteriaceae*, *Pseudomonas*, and gram-positive organisms and is inhibitory for *Listeria* and *Enterococcus faecalis*. The few organisms resistant to it include *Enterococcus faecium*, *Pseudomonas cepacia*, *Corynebacterium jeikeium* (JK), *Xanthomonas maltophilia*, and methicillin-resistant staphylococci. Now about 20% of *P. aeruginosa* are also resistant. Know that imipenem can lower the seizure threshold, so it should only be used as a last resort in seizure patients or in patients with renal insufficiency.

Imipenem is always formulated with equal amounts of cilastatin (combo = Primaxin®). Cilastatin causes metabolism of imipenem to be blocked in the renal tubule thereby increasing its half-life to...one hour! Cilastatin has no effect on beta-lactamases.

Meropenem is a similar carbapenem with a longer half-life so no need for an enzyme inhibitor. It is also less likely to cause seizures than imipenem.

Aztreonam

Aztreonam is a monobactam which is only good against aerobic and facultative gram-negative bacteria. Its spectrum is similar to aminoglycosides (gram-negative aerobes). It is effective against most *Enterobacteriaceae* and against *Pseudomonas* but it is not active against gram-positive cocci or anaerobes.

Beta-lactamase Inhibitors

Beta-lactamase Inhibitors— • sulbactam, • clavulanic acid, and • tazobactam bind irreversibly to the beta-lactamase made by some bacteria. These inhibitors increase the activity of drugs against beta-lactamase producing bacteria such as *B. fragilis*, *Klebsiella*, and *S. aureus* (variably). Formulations:

Clavulanic acid mixed with amoxicillin (Augmentin®, Clavulin®)

Clavulanic acid mixed with ticarcillin (Timentin®)

Sulbactam mixed with ampicillin (Unasyn®)

Tazobactam mixed with piperacillin (Zosyn®, Tazocin®)

OTHER ANTIBIOTICS

Vancomycin

Vancomycin is, in general, bactericidal. It is effective against most gram-positive organisms including methicillin-resistant staphylococci, *Clostridia*, and *Corynebacterium*. There are some vancomycin-resistant strains of enterococci and recent reports of vancomycin-resistant *S. aureus* (yikes!). *Staphylococcus haemolyticus* and a few *Staph epidermidis* are resistant (causing serious trouble in some endocarditis patients!).

Vancomycin sometimes causes the "Red man syndrome" which consists of tachycardia, flushing, occasional angioedema, and generalized pruritus. This can be prevented either by slowing down the infusion time or by pretreatment with antihistamines (but not H2-blockers). Like the aminoglycosides, vancomycin is both oto- and nephrotoxic but to a much lesser degree!

Aminoglycosides

Aminoglycosides are effective against many gram-negative organisms. They require the aerobic mechanism of the cell to be effective, so are no good against anaerobes. Aminoglycosides have a persistent anti-gram-negative effect after removal of the drug—known as the post-antibiotic effect! So it is possible to dose aminoglycosides q24 hours with equivalent or better results than the same daily dosage given more often. Because they irreversibly inhibit ribosomal protein synthesis, they are bactericidal.

Aminoglycosides are effective against *Yersinia pestis* plague (streptomycin), *Francisella tularensis* (streptomycin or gentamicin), *M. tuberculosis* (streptomycin), and *M. avium-intracellulare* (amikacin). Gentamicin is used in combination with a beta-lactam antibiotic for the treatment of subacute bacterial endocarditis. Gentamicin is often given along with rifampin to prevent the rapid development of resistance to rifampin (as in prosthetic valve endocarditis). It is also given to febrile neutropenic patients along with either a third-generation cephalosporin or an antipseudomonal penicillin.

Major side effects of aminoglycoside treatment are ear toxicity and kidney toxicity—these are more likely if either amphotericin B or cephalothin is also used!

Fluoroquinolones

Fluoroquinolones (ciprofloxacin, norfloxacin, ofloxacin, levofloxacin, sparfloxacin, moxifloxacin, gatifloxacin) are a set of very wide spectrum antibiotics which inhibit bacterial DNA synthesis. They are very good against gram-negative aerobic organisms—including rods.

Indications:
- Ciprofloxacin, ofloxacin, and the newer agents can be used for systemic infections.
- Fluoroquinolones are also good against all the usual causes of bacterial gastroenteritis (*Salmonella*, *Shigella*, *Campylobacter*, and *Yersinia enterocolitica*).

Not effective in:
- They are not good against anaerobes (*B. fragilis*, et al).
- Ciprofloxacin and ofloxacin have only intermediate activity against gram-positive organisms, including *S. pneumoniae*. Hence, they are not a good choice for empiric treatment of pneumonia. (On the other hand, levofloxacin, moxifloxacin, and gatifloxacin are alternative choices for community acquired pneumonia. The newer fluoroquinolones are also effective treatment for atypical pneumonias.)
- They are not used for MRSA because of the widespread rapid development of resistance to them.
- They are not given to small children (FDA says no one under 18 years of age) or pregnant patients.

Know: Some fluoroquinolones increase the levels of theophylline and cyclosporine by decreasing metabolism, and increase the effect of warfarin by an uncertain mechanism. They do not increase the elimination of any drug. Although ciprofloxacin and enoxacin, like erythromycin, delay theophylline clearance, norfloxacin and ofloxacin apparently do not.

Macrolides

Erythromycin is a drug to consider for community acquired pneumonia because it is effective against *S. pneumoniae (although increasing resistance)*, *Mycoplasma pneumoniae*, and *Legionella pneumophila*. It is also effective against *Chlamydia pneumoniae*, *Campylobacter* (diarrhea), diphtheria, and pertussis. It is not so good against *H. flu* and is not effective against Q fever (*Coxiella burnetii*) which is treated with tetracycline or chloramphenicol. Like the quinolones, erythromycin increases the effect of theophylline, cyclosporine, and warfarin.

Azithromycin has same indications as erythromycin—and it has better *H. flu* coverage. It has a very long half-life (so once per day dosage) and an intravenous form.

Rifampin is bactericidal. It is never given alone to treat an acute infection because organisms rapidly develop resistance to it.

Oxazolidinones

Oxazolidinones is an entirely new class of antibiotic of which linezolid (Zyvox™) is the first available. They have a unique mechanism of action for the blocking of protein synthesis. The drug binds to the 50S ribosomal subunit thereby preventing attachment of the 30S+mRNA subunit—so the 70S ribosome initiation complex is not made and no protein is produced.

Linezolid is active against gm pos organisms including MRSA (methicillin-resistant *S. aureus*). It is also effective against VRE (vancomycin-resistant enterococci) and anaerobes! Linezolid is available in oral (with 100% bioavailability!) and IV preparations. The oral form makes it a desirable alternative to vancomycin for MRSA—however concerns of developing resistance and cost make this drug an unlikely first line agent.

notes

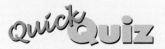
Streptogramins

Quinupristin/dalfopristin (Synercid®) is the first of this new class of antibiotics. It was the first antibiotic approved for the treatment of serious infections with Vancomycin-resistant *Enterococcus faecium*. The main side effects with this antibiotic are its severe myalgias and arthralgias.

ANTIVIRAL AGENTS

Acyclovir is a nucleoside analog used for the treatment of herpes simplex and varicella-zoster viruses. Valacyclovir and famciclovir have similar indications.

Ganciclovir (previously DHPG) is used for the treatment of CMV infections in AIDS patients, especially for the chorioretinitis and colitis. Leukopenia is a side-effect. Because it only has a suppressive effect against CMV, it usually needs to be given until the CD4 lymphocytes are > 200.

Foscarnet is used in patients with ganciclovir-resistant Herpes infection or as an alternative to ganciclovir for CMV.

Ribavirin is indicated for the treatment of RSV and is used as part of combination therapy for Hepatitis C.

Amantadine and rimantadine are effective against influenza A.

Oseltamivir (Tamiflu®—oral) and zanamivir (Relenza®—powder for inhalation) are neuraminidase inhibitors, a new class of treatment for influenza A & B.

See pg 2-25 for the antiretroviral medications.

ANTIFUNGAL AGENTS

Polyenes

There are three major classes of antifungal medicines: polyenes, imidazoles, and triazoles.

• Systemic polyene: Amphotericin B is the standard treatment for most systemic mycoses. Systemic amphotericin B can only be given IV and it has many side effects: fever, renal failure, phlebitis, acidosis, low K+ and Mg. Some recommend giving a test dose first. Every-other-day treatment is just as effective as daily dosage. Hypotension with the first dose may occur (decrease in peripheral vascular tone). Amphotericin B is associated with electrolyte abnormalities—especially hypokalemia, hypomagnesemia, and renal tubular acidosis.

Lipid associated amphotericin B preparations are less nephrotoxic but much more expensive. Use only when toxicity has become a problem with regular amphotericin.

• Topical polyene macrolides: Nystatin and amphotericin topical formulations are only good against cutaneous candidiasis (not ringworm…). Both are also available in liquid form for oral and esophageal candidiasis.

Imidazoles

Systemic imidazole

Ketoconazole for systemic use is given orally—increased gastric pH (low acid) decreases absorption. Absorption is not affected by food. Ketoconazole does not penetrate CSF well. It is occasionally used for palliative treatment of Cushing syndrome caused by ectopic production of ACTH (i.e., cancer) because it blocks the 11-hydroxylase enzyme in the adrenal gland, thereby decreasing the amount of cortisol produced (more in the Endocrinology section).

Ketoconazole increases levels of indinavir and digoxin and potentiates benzodiazepines. Side effects of ketoconazole include nausea and hepatitis. It also causes a decrease in androgen production, so patients may have decreased libido and males may get gynecomastia.

Ketoconazole is cheaper than fluconazole or itraconazole but has largely been replaced by them for serious fungal infections. It has many interactions with common drugs—sometimes dangerous.

Topical imidazoles:

Clotrimazole and miconazole are available in both cutaneous and vaginal preparations. Other cutaneous imidazoles are ketoconazole, econazole, sulconazole, and oxiconazole. Other vaginal formulations are butoconazole and tioconazole. Spectrum and efficacy is the same. All are effective in the treatment of cutaneous candidiasis, tinea versicolor, and ringworm.

Triazoles

Systemic triazoles:

Itraconazole is a triazole analogue of ketoconazole and is generally more effective and safer. The liquid formulation has much better bioavailability. Food enhances absorption. Indications are the same as ketoconazole (histoplasmosis, blastomycosis, coccidioidomycosis, esophageal candidiasis, and chronic mucocutaneous candidiasis) but also include aspergillosis, cryptococcosis, sporotrichosis, and onychomycosis.

Fluconazole (Diflucan®). Main side effect is N/V. A single 150 mg oral dose is effective in vulvovaginal candidiasis! Fluconazole is also effective treatment for oral and esophageal candidiasis and candidemia. It has excellent penetration into the CSF and it is often used for maintenance therapy in AIDS patients with cryptococcal meningitis—after an initial 2 week course of IV amphotericin B. Fluconazole is the treatment of choice for chronic coccidioidomycosis.

notes

Topical triazoles:

There is only one vaginal formulation: <u>terconazole</u>.

Other Antifungals
Other systemic antifungals:

Flucytosine (5-fluorocytosine; 5-FC) is highly soluble and penetrates well into the CSF. Upon entering a fungal cell, it is metabolized to the antimetabolite 5-fluorouracil. If used alone, drug resistance develops quickly. For this reason and because it may have a synergistic antifungal effect with amphotericin B, it is combined with amphotericin B to treat cryptococcosis and serious forms of candidiasis. It can cause serious GI, hepatic, renal, and bone marrow toxicities—the latter usually presents as neutropenia and thrombocytopenia. Slight decreases in renal function can increase 5-FC to toxic levels.

Caspofungin acetate (Cancidas®) is the first of a new class of drugs called echinocandins—a glucan synthesis inhibitor. It is approved for invasive aspergillosis in severely immuno-compromised patients.

Other topical antifungals:

Undecylenic acid and tolnaftate are effective only against ringworm. The following cutaneous preparations have the same efficacy and clinical spectrum as the imidazoles: naftifine, terbinafine, haloprogin, and ciclopirox olamine.

ANTIPARASITIC DRUGS

Praziquantel (Biltricide®, outstanding drug) is the only drug effective against all species of *Schistosoma* and so is the drug of choice for schistosomiasis. It is also good against flukes and tapeworms (i.e., used to treat neurocysticercosis—caused by the pork tapeworm, *T. solium*).
Albendazole is now used for cysticercosis and schistosomiasis. (pg 2-20)
Niclosamide is also used for the treatment of tapeworm but it affects only those in the intestine.
Pentamidine, which is used for treatment (IV form) and for the prophylaxis (inhaled form) of *Pneumocystis carinii* (which is most likely a fungus), has many side effects including azotemia (1/4), leukopenia, pancreatitis, and hypo- or hyperglycemia. It causes no significant skin reactions.
Anti-malaria drugs. See pg 2-18.

VACCINES

For Vaccines, see "Preventive Medicine" in the General Internal Medicine section.

BACTERIA
GRAM-POSITIVE ORGANISMS

Staph aureus causes bacteremia especially among IV drug users and dialysis patients. It is also a cause of toxic shock syndrome (TSS) and the cause of toxic epidermal necrolysis (scalded skin syndrome). Pathogenicity (which is not the same as resistance to antibiotics!) is associated with production of entero- and exotoxin, coagulase, and leukocidin. In chronic carriers, *S. aureus* is found on the nasal mucosa cultures but not in the blood.
The percentage of methicillin-resistant *S. aureus* (MRSA) infections has grown substantially due to indiscriminate use of methicillin and similar antibiotics. In most hospitals, 15-20% of *S. aureus* isolates are MRSA. In some tertiary care centers, the percentage is over 50%! Unfortunately, MRSA is now frequently seen in community acquired infections as well!
In carriers, it is difficult to eradicate—can try topical mupirocin ointment (Bactroban®) and oral rifampin but, even then, it still recurs. In all cases of bacteremia and serious infection with MRSA, vancomycin is the ONLY drug of choice. Although other drugs may be used for their synergistic effect (gentamicin and rifampin), vancomycin is always required. In some skin and soft tissue infections, other antibiotics may be effective including TMP/SMX or clindamycin, each +/– rifampin. There is rapidly developing resistance against quinolones.
More on toxic shock. TSS often presents with red skin, hypotension, fever, diarrhea, and hypocalcemia. With young women, TSS is usually associated with menstruation and tampon use. A young woman with the focus in the uterus may have a bloody discharge or be menstruating. The hypocalcemia is not treated unless either symptoms or ECG signs develop. Any time there is a post-surgical toxic shock, any device implanted during the surgery must be immediately removed (prosthetic device, implant, etc.).
Another cause of TSS is *Streptococcus pyogenes*. This usually results from a progressive skin infection—especially post-op and with chickenpox! Note that in staph TSS, blood cultures are usually negative; whereas in strep TSS, blood cultures are usually positive!
Staphylococcus is the usual cause of furuncles and carbuncles [pg 8, #24].

S. epidermidis and *S. saprophyticus* are examples of coagulase-negative *Staph*. *Staph epi* is almost always methicillin resistant. It is the most common cause of both catheter-related bacteremia (catheter gets contaminated as it passes through the skin) and bacteremia occurring post-op when anything foreign was left in the body (prosthetics, including heart valves and joints, pacemakers, shunts etc.). Treat with vancomycin +/- rifampin +/- gentamicin. *S. saprophyticus* causes UTI in young women.

Streptococcus pneumoniae—Remember: you need functioning spleen and antibodies to defend against the encapsulated *S. pneumoniae* and *H. influenzae*—so both infections are seen

notes

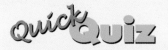

more often in splenectomized patients (including those with SS disease), very young and old patients, and in CLL, MM, and agammaglobulinemia (i.e., any antibody dysfunction or decrease). Alcoholics also are more susceptible, but not because of antibody problems.

About 30% of *S. pneumoniae* have developed some degree of resistance to penicillin. For serious infections (e.g., meningitis or bacteremia) use ceftriaxone until PCN sensitivity is known. For high-level resistance, vancomycin should be used. For meningitis with high-level penicillin resistance, use ceftriaxone and vancomycin. For outpatients allergic to PCN, give doxycycline, cephalosporin, macrolide, or quinolone.

Remember: postsplenectomy pneumococcal sepsis can be rapidly fatal and can present with flu-like symptoms, purpura, and DIC (test question will have Howell-Jolly bodies on peripheral smear).

S. pyogenes is the only species in Group A, beta-hemolytic strep. It may cause strep pharyngitis, streptococcal TSS, rheumatic fever, and scarlet fever [pg 9, #26]. The major protein on its cell surface is the "M protein." The M protein occurs in over 80 antigenically distinct types and defines which strains are rheumatogenic, cause glomerulonephritis, toxigenic for toxic shock syndrome, etc.

Strep pharyngitis (usually *S. pyogenes*) is more likely with each of these three findings: temp > 100°, tender cervical lymphadenopathy, and exudative tonsils. If none of these are found, chance of *Strep* is < 3%; one = 20%; three = 50%. Again: with strep TSS, blood cultures are usually positive; whereas with staph TSS, blood cultures are usually negative.

On the other hand, if a person comes in with tonsillitis, swollen cervical nodes, and fever but a negative strep test, do you treat with antibiotics? No! What else gives you these symptoms? Think upper respiratory viruses, mononucleosis, and don't forget acute retroviral syndrome (pg 2-29)!

Strep agalactiae (Group B) is seen in the very young and old, especially if the elderly patients are alcoholic or diabetic. It is a major cause of newborn pneumonia and meningitis (this is why ampicillin is included in the empiric treatment for meningitis in the elderly or neonates). It is associated with UTIs in pregnant women and it is also a cause of postpartum endometritis and bacteremia. It can originate from a GU reservoir. Treat with PCN or ampicillin.

Enterococcus faecalis causes 85% of enterococcal infections while *Enterococcus faecium* causes 15%. The source of these organisms is usually either the GI or urinary tract. Suspect an enterococcal infection if a patient gets sepsis and/or endocarditis after a TURP.

All enterococci are resistant to all cephalosporins and penicillinase-resistant penicillins, and moderately resistant to the aminoglycosides. *E. faecium* is one of the few organisms resistant to imipenem and is causing great problems with rapidly emerging strong resistance to vancomycin ("VRE").

If sensitive, vancomycin, PCN, and ampicillin are only inhibitory but!... an aminoglycoside in combination with any of these is effective treatment. So... sensitive enterococcal sepsis or endocarditis must be treated with vancomycin, PCN, or ampicillin in addition to gentamicin. Resistance to these antibiotics is increasing so it is imperative that you do sensitivity testing.

Listeria monocytogenes infections are associated with decreased cellular immunity syndromes like AIDS, lymphoma, and leukemia but they are also seen in neonates, the elderly, and pregnant women. For some reason it is not actually seen as much as expected in AIDS patients. Mortality rate in listerial meningitis is 30% overall.

Like enterococcus, *Listeria* is resistant to all cephalosporins (again, this is why ampicillin is included in the empiric treatment for meningitis in the elderly or neonates). Also, as with the enterococci, PCN and ampicillin are only inhibitory but!... an aminoglycoside in combination with either of these is very effective treatment.

Even so, most mild to moderate cases of listeriosis do not require an aminoglycoside but treat resistant or serious cases with PCN or ampicillin in combination with an aminoglycoside. Vancomycin or TMP/SMX if allergic to PCN. Because aminoglycosides do not penetrate the CSF well, very high dose PCN or ampicillin is used to treat listerial meningitis. Again:

• Mild to moderate listeriosis: Amp
• Serious/resistant: Amp + aminoglycoside
• Listerial meningitis: high dose Amp +/- aminoglycoside

Corynebacterium diphtheriae causes diphtheria [pg 11, #32]. Diphtheria is an upper respiratory infection with a gray-white pharyngeal membrane, hoarseness, sore throat, and a low fever (< 101°)! Low fever! Toxic effects include myocarditis with possible cardiac failure and polyneuritis. Treatment is erythromycin. Second choice is penicillin. Diphtheria antitoxin is always given with the antibiotic.

notes

Corynebacterium jeikeium (JK) is especially a problem in neutropenic patients and in bone marrow transplant units where it is a cause of IV catheter-related infections. It is resistant to most drugs. Vancomycin is the only effective agent.

Arcanobacterium haemolyticum (previously *Corynebacterium haemolyticum*) causes a pharyngitis similar to that of *Strep pyogenes* with a desquamative scarlatiniform rash and lymphadenitis. It is effectively treated with PCN, erythromycin, or tetracycline.

Bacillus anthracis are large gram-positive rods (bacilli) which cause anthrax. There are two types of anthrax: cutaneous (95% [pg 10, #29]) and pulmonic ("woolsorters disease"). Recent bioterrorist attacks have made this organism appear on the Boards! Know it! Inoculation occurs from handling contaminated hides/wool or (recently) mail. Cutaneous form starts as a painless papule that vesiculates and forms a painless ulcer and then a painless black eschar, often with a lot of nonpitting, painless induration and swelling. *B. anthracis* produces a tripartite exotoxin, consisting of edema factor, protective antigen, and lethal factor. Both edema factor and lethal factor require protective antigen to be active. Treatment of choice for both types of anthrax is penicillin G. Second choice may be tetracycline, or a quinolone.

Bacillus cereus is a close relative of *Bacillus anthracis*. Endotoxin-producing strains cause gastroenteritis of two varieties: 1) a short incubation (1-6 hr) emetic type and a longer incubation (8-16 hr) diarrheal type. Like *S. aureus*, the endotoxin is produced outside the host and therefore has a quick onset of symptoms (1-6 hr). The emetic form is associated with fried rice left at room temperature for awhile. This gastroenteritis is self-limited and necessitates only symptomatic treatment. It is an occasional cause of infection in contact lens wearers, after a traumatic eye injury, and is a possible cause of IV catheter-related infections. Treatment for serious disease is vancomycin.

Clostridium is a strict anaerobic gram-positive rod.
- *C. difficile* causes antibiotic-associated colitis (see pg 2-35).
- *C. botulinum* causes botulism—this toxin is the most potent known! It blocks presynaptic acetylcholine release.
- *C. perfringens* is one of the most common causes of food poisoning in the U.S.
- *C. septicum*: The majority of patients with *C. septicum* sepsis have an associated GI malignancy!
- *C. tetani* is the cause of tetanus [pg 11, #31].

Cellulitis and gas gangrene can be caused by *C. septicum, perfringens, tetani*, or *novyi* [pg 10, #30]. The main toxin in all *Clostridia* is the "alpha toxin." For acute antibiotic treatment of *C. tetani* and *C. perfringens*, use PCN (tetracycline or clindamycin if allergic). For tetanus also remember to use tetanus toxoid and tetanus immune globulin! Look for it an elderly person with lock-jaw!

Gram-positive and gram-negative beta-lactamase producing bacteria: *Staphylococcus* (most), *N. gonorrhoeae* and *H. influenzae* (25%), *Enterobacteriaceae, M. catarrhalis, B. fragilis.*

GRAM-NEG BACTERIA

Neisseria meningitidis is a gram-negative coccus which is an occasional ordinary inhabitant of the human throat. It usually does not cause disease because specific antibodies (humoral defense) and complement lyse the organisms as they enter the bloodstream.

Patients with complement deficiency are especially prone to meningococcemia. Meningococcemia presents with fever, hypotension, diffuse purpuric lesions, and DIC (for more on DIC, see Hematology section). [pg 10, #28]

Penicillin G is the treatment of choice; for the penicillin-allergic, give fluoroquinolones (to adults) or 3rd generation cephalosporins (if rash only) to child. With prompt treatment, the mortality rate of meningococcemia is 10%. Rifampin or fluoroquinolones are better for eradicating the carrier state because they concentrate in the throat mucosa.

Neisseria gonorrhoeae is a common cause of sexually transmitted disease. It is a gram-negative organism which is usually found as diplococci. The penicillinase-producing strains of *N. gonorrhoeae* now account for 50% of cases in many areas in Asia and Africa and are also common in the U.S.. More on pg 2-36.

Moraxella catarrhalis (formerly *Branhamella catarrhalis* [formerly *Neisseria catarrhalis*!]) is a gram-negative coccus which causes respiratory infections, especially in immunodeficient patients and patients with COPD. It is a common cause of sinusitis in adults and otitis media in children. Treat adults with amoxicillin/clavulanate, 2nd or 3rd generation cephalosporin, or a quinolone. In the U.S., almost all are susceptible to erythromycin, tetracycline, and TMP/SMX.

Pseudomonas aeruginosa is a small gram-negative rod with a single flagellum. *Pseudomonas aeruginosa* is suggested if there is a history of nail-puncture wounds (especially if through a tennis shoe), osteomyelitis and endocarditis in IV drug abusers, and chronic otitis externa (which can be especially severe in diabetics). Ecthyma gangrenosum (round indurated black lesion with central ulceration) is seen with pseudomonal bacteremia. *Pseudomonas* is the cause of "hot tub rash" which people get from improperly chlorinated hot tubs (this is usually self-limited).

Enterobacteriaceae is a family which are gram-negative enteric bacilli and include: *Salmonella, Yersinia, Shigella, Citrobacter*, and *Edwardsiella*.

Salmonella are gram-negative bacilli which are usually motile. Non-typhoidal salmonella are a fairly common cause of diarrhea. Because the bacteria are not host-adapted like *S. typhi*, they can be found in many different nonhuman host animals. It may be spread by frozen foods (especially chicken), milk, and eggs. Baby chicks, iguanas, turtles, and other exotic pets

notes

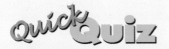

may also be sources of infections. Treatment increases the risk of developing a carrier state.

Salmonella typhi is, unlike most *Salmonella,* non-motile and encapsulated. It causes typhoid fever, usually from contaminated food, milk, or water. Adults are more likely to be carriers because *S. typhi* tends to seed in gallstones (did "typhoid Mary" have gallstones?). The infection tends to cause *leukopenia.* The classic "rose spots" form on the trunk about a *week* after the fever starts; these look like little 2-3 mm diameter angiomas [pg 14, #40].

Typhoid vaccine is recommended for travelers (> 2 years old) who go outside of the usual tourist areas of Latin America, Asia, and Africa—it is covered in the Preventive Medicine section.

Treatment of typhoid fever: options include quinolones, 3rd generation cephalosporins, ampicillin, TMP/SMX, and chloramphenicol depending on sensitivities. Carriers without gallbladder disease or stones can usually be cleared with 6 weeks of ampicillin + probenecid. (The probenecid decreases clearance and causes a higher blood level of the ampicillin.)

Yersinia pestis is a gram-negative coccobacillus which causes plague. Reservoir is wild rodents. It is transmitted by fleas or direct contact (skinning animals, high mortality). The bubonic type causes large localized lymphadenopathy ("buboes") that suppurates. If not treated, it can lead to sepsis and death. The bubonic type also may lead to a pulmonic form which is rapidly transmitted to bystanders by coughing. (Again bioterrorism has brought this organism back to the exam of the ABIM!) Note that plague and tularemia present similarly (adenopathy after hunting etc.) except the geographic locations are different—desert SW for plague versus Arkansas, Missouri, and Oklahoma for tularemia.

Diagnosis of plague is made by aspirating the lymph nodes.

Treat plague with streptomycin. Second line choices: tetracycline or quinolones.

Other *Enterobacteriaceae* are covered under diarrhea in the GI section.

The Legionellaceae family comprises many species—of which *Legionella pneumophila* causes 80-90% of human Legionellaceae infections. Legionellaceae are aerobic gram-negative bacilli which require a particular media to grow.

Legionella is contained in water and modes of transmission are multiple—with aspiration as the most likely.

Legionella pneumophila infection (legionellosis) causes legions of problems. Multisystem disease is the clue! Patients often have diarrhea and CNS symptoms (H/A, delirium, and *confusion*) presenting in addition to the pneumonia. Presentation is similar to, and often confused with, *Mycoplasma pneumoniae.* Like *M. pneumoniae,* the CXR is much worse looking than the exam indicates.

Treatment for moderate infections is azithromycin—or quinolones. If severely ill, rifampin is added.

Klebsiella and other gram-negative causes of pneumonia are in the Pulmonary section.

Brucellosis is a zoonosis caused by an aerobic gram-negative bacillus which, worldwide, is usually caused by *B. melitensis* (goats, sheep, and camels). Other strains: *Brucella abortus* (cattle), *B. suis* (pigs), and *B. canis* (dogs). It is often transmitted to humans via unpasteurized milk or cheese or by inhalation (work-related). It affects the heart (especially suspect in culture-negative endocarditis), lungs, GI tract, GU (orchitis, abortion), and endocrine glands (thyroiditis, adrenal insufficiency, SIADH). Check for brucellosis in a FUO workup! Confirming the diagnosis is difficult. Cultures may take up to 6 weeks to grow. In some types serotyping (looking for increasing specific IgM titers) can be done.

Treatment requires combination therapy:
doxycycline + aminoglycoside (streptomycin, gentamicin, or netilmicin) x 4 wks or
doxycycline + rifampin x 4-8 wks.

Quinolones are effective for acute disease but may have a higher relapse rate.

Francisella tularensis is a small, gram-negative pleomorphic bacillus which causes tularemia ("rabbit fever"). It is found in many animals. It is transmitted by ticks and blood-sucking flies but the organism may also be ingested or inhaled. Especially seen in Arkansas, Missouri, and Oklahoma. Typically, patients with tularemia present with a history of sudden onset of fever, chills, myalgias, and arthralgias followed by an irregular ulcer at the site of inoculation which may persist for months. Regional lymphadenopathy develops and these nodes may necrose and suppurate.

Diagnosis of tularemia is based on the typical clinical syndrome and is confirmed with serologic testing for *Francisella tularensis.* Differential includes plague which occurs mostly in the desert SW.

Treat with streptomycin, gentamicin or tetracycline if not severely ill.

notes

Bartonella bacilliformis causes bartonellosis, a disease which has two manifestations—severe/acute and chronic. Bartonella are <u>tiny gram-negative pleomorphic</u> bacteria. It is transmitted by sandflies only in the Andes mountains (Peru etc.). The only known reservoir is humans.

The initial, acute form consists of rapid onset of a febrile hemolytic anemia with a high mortality if untreated (50%)! This is called "Oroya fever." The chronic benign form with chronic cutaneous lesions is called "verruga peruana." *Salmonella* is a common cause of coinfection with Oroya fever. (Hmm! just as in the hemolytic anemia of SS disease).

Oroya fever usually responds dramatically to tetracycline or chloramphenicol. Chloramphenicol is preferred because it also is effective against *Salmonella*.

Bartonella henselae causes cat-scratch disease or, in the immunocompromised patient, bacillary angiomatosis. The skin lesions of bacillary angiomatosis are identical to "verruga peruana" (above). Treatment: erythromycin +/- rifampin depending on severity. Recent data support the use of azithromycin for treatment of cat-scratch disease. Note: do not biopsy nodes.

Helicobacter pylori is a gram-negative spiral flagellated bacillus. It causes gastritis and PUD and is a risk factor for adenocarcinoma of the stomach. Discussed in Gastroenterology section.

RICKETTSIAL

Rickettsia rickettsii, a <u>gram-negative coccobacillus,</u> causes <u>Rocky Mountain spotted fever</u> (RMSF)—know! This disease has a 3% mortality. Classic signs and symptoms include a rash, fever, arthralgias (but *not* overt arthritis), and a history of recent exposure to ticks. The rash occurs on the distal extremities. It progresses from maculopapular to petechial. Most infected persons get the rash but few get all the classic signs and symptoms. Patients may also present with diarrhea and abdominal pain.

Most clinicians diagnose this on clinical grounds, start treatment, and then confirm with serological testing. For a definite diagnosis, do immunofluorescent staining on a biopsy of the petechial lesion.

Other rickettsial infections include *R. typhi* (<u>endemic typhus</u>), *R. prowazekii* (<u>epidemic typhus</u>), *R. conorii* (<u>Mediterranean spotted fever</u>), and *Coxiella burnetii* (<u>Q fever</u>). Know that Q fever is a zoonosis which is transmitted to humans mainly by inhalation of the aerosol released from the infected animal. Q fever is seen in abattoir (slaughterhouse) workers and in people exposed to an infected animal's products of conception during birthing. Buzzwords: Cattle or Cats + Cilled (☹!) or Conception = Coxiella (Q fever).

Treat **all** *Rickettsia* infections with tetracycline/doxycycline or chloramphenicol. Quinolones may also be effective. Vaccines have no effect.

Ehrlichia infection (ehrlichiosis) has been called "spotless Rocky Mountain Fever". There are two forms of the disease:

1) "<u>Human Monocytic Ehrlichiosis</u>" (HME) and <u>Human Granulocytic Ehrlichiosis</u> (HGE). The organism is small, gram-negative, and obligately intracellular. HME is due to *E. chaffeensis* and mainly seen in Missouri and Arkansas while HGE is likely due to either *E. phagocytophilia* or *E. equi* and predominates in the northeast and midwest. There is usually no rash. The organism affects the monocytes or neutrophils and patients typically present with the viral picture of fever, headache, and leukopenia, and they may also have thrombocytopenia. Think of this in a presentation of pancytopenia and tick-bite! Treatment is doxycycline/tetracycline.

Note: there are reports of dual infection with *Ehrlichia + Babesia microti* (an intra-RBC protozoan parasite) and *Ehrlichia + Borrelia burgdorferi* (Lyme) in the endemic northeast areas.

GRAM-VARIABLE

<u>*Gardnerella vaginalis*</u> (previously called *Haemophilus vaginalis*) is gram variable. Treat with metronidazole. It is associated with a vaginosis. More on pg 2-37.

ACID-FAST

All *Mycobacteria* are acid-fast (red on a green background). Pleural effusions associated with *M. tuberculosis* have a lymphocyte count of 1,000-6,000/mm^3, a low glucose, elevated protein, and elevated LDH. The glucose is normally > 80 although, in 20% of cases, it is < 60.

• *M. scrofulaceum* and *M. avium-intracellulare* cause lymphadenitis in children; treat by excising the nodes!

• *M. leprae* causes leprosy [pg 13, #38-39]. Transmission is probably via respiratory droplets person-to-person. Diagnose with Fite stains of skin or nerve.

• *M. marinum* is the "fish-tank bacillus." It causes nonhealing skin ulceration in people working around fish tanks. It often causes strings of lesions along the lymphatic channels. Treat *M. marinum* with ethambutol + rifampin or clarithromycin + rifampin (more on pg 2-38).

• TB is covered in the Pulmonary section.

Nocardia asteroides is only weakly acid-fast (easily missed). Its shape is beaded, branching, and filamentous. It usually starts as a lung infection—occasionally causing a thin-walled cavitary lesion. It can cause focal brain abscesses and a neutrophilic chronic meningitis (most chronic meningitides are lymphocytic). Nodular skin lesions are common. It is hard to isolate.

Usual treatment is with high-dose sulfonamides or TMP/SMX. In severely ill patients combinations of drugs are added including Amikacin + imipenem. Minocycline is another alternate choice for those sulfa allergic.

Nocardia brasiliensis is in the soil. Like *M. marinum*, it can cause inflammation with associated surface lesions along lymphatic channels. Treat with sulfonamides or TMP/SMX.

notes

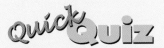
Resistant to imipenem (*N. asteroides* is sensitive to imipenem).

Cryptosporidium and *Isospora belli* are both acid-fast and both are common causes of chronic diarrhea in AIDS patients. The *Isospora* are large and oval shaped; treat infection with TMP/SMX. Infection with *Cryptosporidia* (which are small and round) is usually self-limited in immunocompetent patients and requires no treatment. In immunocompromised patients people have tried paromomycin and albendazole with varying success.

OTHER ORGANISMS

Actinomyces is an anaerobic organism which causes an infection in which there grows characteristic yellow "sulfur" granules which are actually clusters of organisms. The usual presentation of actinomycosis is cervicofacial involvement caused by a dental infection [pg 11, #33]. Actinomyces is a cause of PID when there is an IUD in place. It occasionally causes a chronic neutrophilic meningitis (as do *Nocardia* and fungi). Treatment is PCN or ampicillin. Second choice is tetracycline.

Chlamydia are obligate intracellular parasites. C. *psittaci*, C. *trachomatis,* and C. *pneumonia* (formerly TWAR) are pathogenic in humans.
- *C. psittaci is* found in psittacine and other birds and causes psittacosis: pneumonia and *splenomegaly. Again:* any pneumonia associated with poultry, especially with splenomegaly, strongly suggests *C. psittaci* (DDx: *Histoplasma also* causes pneumonia and splenomegaly; it is associated with bird and bat droppings). Onset of psittacosis is associated with myalgias, rigors, headache, and high fever—to 105°F.
- *C pneumonia* (TWAR) causes community-acquired pneumonia in adults who have not been exposed to birds, i.e., person-to-person spread. Bronchospasm is particularly prominent in respiratory infection caused by *C. pneumonia.*

- *C. trachomatis* causes the GU infections and trachoma (chronic external eye infection causing cataracts, but not glaucoma; it is found especially in Asia and Africa). Approximately 5% of pregnant women have *Chlamydia trachomatis* in their genital tracts; antibiotic ointment in infants' eyes at birth prevents the conjunctivitis. The same *C. trachomatis* is also associated with neonatal pneumonia! Lymphogranuloma venereum is an STD caused by the same *C trachomatis,* but a different immunotype.

ETC...

Sepsis is associated with an elevated WBC with left shift, increased PT and PTT, and metabolic acidosis but overwhelming sepsis can cause leukopenia. Gram-negative septic shock is associated with warm extremities because, despite the decreased blood pressure, there is no compensatory peripheral vasoconstriction (i.e., peripheral vascular resistance numbers are low). Cardiac index is elevated (normal is 2.8-4.2 L/min/m^2).

Antibiotic prophylaxis is recommended for procedures associated with high risk of infection (such as hysterectomies both vaginal and abdominal and bowel surgeries), procedures involving implantation of prosthetic material (such as joint replacement), and some procedures when infections, if they occur, would be especially serious (Cardiothoracic). The drug of choice almost always is Cefazolin!

Staph, Salmonella, and *Serratia* are more likely to be seen in patients with granulomatous disease. And again, *H. influenzae, S. pneumoniae,* and meningococci are more likely in patients with spleen or antibody dysfunction. For dysfunctional T-cell associated infections, see AIDS-associated infections on pg 2-29. *Aspergillus, Mucor,* and *Pseudomonas* infections are more likely in granulocytopenic patients (leukemia, chemotherapy, post transplant) than in AIDS patients.

SPIROCHETES
SYPHILIS

Syphilis is caused by *Treponema pallidum.* Sequence of infection:

- <u>Primary</u> syphilis has diffuse metastases with a painless chancre within 3-40 days (depending on the number of inoculating organisms) and regional lymphadenopathy. In women, if the infection is cervical, it is often asymptomatic. Chancre lasts 2-6 weeks and then resolves.
- <u>Secondary</u> syphilis occurs about 2 months later with generalized lymphadenopathy, constitutional symptoms, and mucosal (35%) or cutaneous (90%) lesions that can mimic many other lesions ("the great imitator"). The skin lesions may be macular or papular but are rarely vesicular. They can occur on the palms and soles. These signs and symptoms resolve in 3-12 weeks and the disease goes into a la-

notes

tency period. Untreated, 1/3 of secondary syphilis cases eventually proceed to tertiary syphilis.

- Tertiary syphilis: CNS lues ("lues" is just another word for syphilis), aortitis (aneurysm rupture is the main cause of death from syphilis!), and tabes dorsalis (causes demyelination, resulting in foot-slap and a wide-based gait). One CNS manifestation is the Argyll Robertson pupil [pg 159, #476], which is miotic (small) and irregular; it reacts normally to accommodation (contracts when focusing close, dilates when focusing on distant objects) but not to light.

Serology. There are two general types of tests: nontreponemal/reagin (VDRL and RPR) and specific Treponemal (MHA-TP and FTA-ABS tests. 20-30% of patients with primary syphilis are negative by either type of test but will turn positive shortly thereafter. 99-100% of patients will be positive by either test in secondary syphilis. Once positive, the specific treponemal tests (MHA-TP and FTA-ABS) stay positive for life. The nontreponemal tests become negative after treatment unless treatment has been delayed for many years, in which case they may stay positive.

Scenarios (know):

1) –RPR +MHA-TP:
   a) Successfully treated for syphilis in the past or
   b) early infection or
   c) false positive—see below. Check for history of Lyme disease and repeat RPR in 6 weeks.

2) +RPR –MHA-TP:
   a) Probably early infection or
   b) often a false positive in low risk population. Repeat in 6 weeks.

3) +RPR, +MHA-TP: Infection

Antibodies to *Borrelia burgdorferi* (Lyme) cross-react and may cause a false-positive treponemal test (MHA-TP and FTA-ABS) but does not affect a nontreponemal test (VDRL and RPR).

If the VDRL or RPR becomes negative after treatment, it is a good indication of successful treatment. The nontreponemal tests may become negative in untreated persons with tertiary syphilis. So, secondary syphilis can typically be screened out by either test being negative, only the treponemal test can be used to screen out tertiary syphilis. I do not say "rule out" because, unfortunately, the false negative rate in tertiary syphilis with the reagin (nontreponemal) tests is up to 30%!

All pregnant women should get a nontreponemal test in the 1st trimester. If at high risk, it should be repeated in the 3rd trimester and at delivery.

Note that all the standard antibody tests in a newborn are positive if the mother was positive, because of crossover of IgG. The previously used newborn IgM test was not very sensitive because the maternal IgG tends to "overwhelm" IgM response.

Note: More sensitive and specific newborn IgM tests are used to check for *Toxoplasma*, rubella, and CMV.

Treatment of syphilis:

For primary syphilis and for the early latency period of secondary syphilis (< 1 year since acquiring the disease) is

- benzathine PCN G 2.4 MU IM or doxycycline 100 mg bid for 14 days.

Late latency secondary syphilis and tertiary syphilis with gummas or cardiovascular problems are treated with

- benzathine PCN G 2.4 MU IM q week x 3 or doxycycline 100 mg PO bid x 4 weeks.

For neurosyphilis, the patient is treated with

- PCN G 18-24 MU IV qd for 10-14 days. This is sometimes followed by benzathine PCN 2.4 MU IM qwk x 3. An alternative is procaine PCN 2.4 MU IM qd with probenecid 500 mg qid for 14 days. If PCN allergic, the best course is to desensitize the patient according to CDC protocol and give the PCN. Ceftriaxone can be used as an alternative for PCN allergic patients with 2 grams a day for 10-14 days. Oral doxycycline is NOT effective for neurosyphilis.

Pregnant women and newborns are treated for syphilis only with PCN. If the pregnant woman is PCN-allergic, she should be desensitized and then treated with PCN. After treatment, a quantitative nontreponemal/reagin test should be done q month while pregnant.

This is the procedure with newborns with possible syphilis:

- If the mother was ineffectively treated, not treated with PCN, treated less than 4 weeks before delivery, or there is a clinical suspicion, the newborn should be treated with PCN.
- If treatment of the mother was sufficient, follow the infant's physical examination, CSF exam and nontreponemal serologic titers—and treat if there is a rise in titer or other abnormality.

Non-venereal treponemal diseases include yaws, pinta, and bejel.

LEPTOSPIROSIS

Leptospirosis is a spirochetal disease transferred by contact with infected animals or contaminated water. It is considered to be the most wide-spread zoonosis in the world. It causes a wide range of symptoms from myalgias, fever, and headache with or without aseptic meningitis to Weil's syndrome: severe hepatitis with renal failure and hemorrhagic complications (renal or hepatic symptoms may predominate). Pulmonary symptoms are also common. The hepatitis is characterized by the bilirubin being disproportionately elevated compared to the liver enzymes. The variety of presenting symptoms makes for a high incidence of initial misdiagnosis. Clue: Look for contact with dog or rat urine. Treat with PCN or doxycycline.

LYME DISEASE

Borrelia burgdorferi causes Lyme disease. It is transmitted by the *Ixodes scapularis (previously Ixodes dammini)* tick in the Northeast and the *Ixodes pacificus* tick in the California area. The protozoa *Babesia is also transmitted by Ixodes scapulars*—see pg 2-19. Lyme disease is generally thought to be

notes

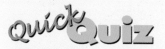

confined to the Northeast but it actually can be found in virtually all the lower 48 states. Saying that, if you practice in Arkansas or Missouri, Ehrlichiosis is much more common than Lyme disease. The *I. scapularis* tick seems to be a better vector so the disease is seen most frequently in the Northeast, especially Martha's Vineyard and the Nantucket area. It does cross the placenta and causes fetal infection and death.

For the most part, ticks transmit Lyme disease during the nymph stage, probably because nymphs are more likely to feed on a person and are rarely noticed because of their small size (less than 2 mm). Thus, the nymphs typically have ample time to feed and transmit the infection (ticks are most likely to transmit infection after approximately 2 or more days of feeding). If a person says they had a tick on them for an hour or two the previous day, just reassure them that no treatment is necessary.

Diagnosis is clinical: erythema chronicum migrans (ECM) is the pathognomonic skin lesion of the early Stage I disease; it starts at the site of the bite and is a slowly spreading irregular erythematous lesion with a clear center [pg 15, #43]. Other early symptoms include myalgias, arthralgias, fever, HA, and lymphadenopathy. Then, weeks to months later, Stage II disease occurs with recurring erythema chronicum migrans (rare), neurologic problems (lymphocytic meningitis and/or neuritis), and heart problems (myocarditis which may cause a rapidly alternating first, second, or third degree AV block). The neuritis often presents as a peripheral neuropathy or a cranial nerve palsy [pg 160, #479-485] or both; consider it in a patient with a suggestive history and Bell's palsy or foot drop or both. Months to years later, Stage III occurs with, most commonly, arthritis (oligo- or migratory—small or large joints—usually large) but there can also be chronic neurologic syndromes. A definite diagnosis may be difficult to establish. Serology is negative in 90% of Stage I so the diagnosis is based on clinical findings. Note: They will give you a patient with ery-thema chronicum migrans—they then ask you do you want to check Lyme serology? The answer is NO! Just Treat! Lyme authorities recommend for patients living in endemic areas who present with recurrent oligoarticular inflammatory arthritis to do an ELISA followed by a Western blot and treat patients with positive results by either test.

Early disease and Bell's palsy are treated with oral doxycycline 100mg bid or amoxicillin for 21 days. Lyme arthritis is treated initially with oral agents as above and then are re-treated with the same oral agent or ceftriaxone if no response initially. Non-responders frequently are HLA-DR4 allele positive. Cardiac and neurologic sequelae are treated with ceftriaxone 2gms or PCN G 20 MU IV x 21 days. No prophylaxis is indicated—i.e., medications are not given prior to camping out or for tick bites.

There was a recombinant outer surface protein (OspA) Lyme disease vaccine (LYMErix®), but it was pulled from the market.

NOTE: For a patient they present to you with fatigue, joint stiffness (not arthritis), muscular aches and/or tenderness: DO NOT CHECK LYME TITERS AND DO NOT TREAT FOR LYME BASED ON THESE NON-SPECIFIC FINDINGS!

Other *Borrelia* infections are *B. recurrentis* and *B. vincentii* which cause relapsing fever (in this, spirochetes are seen in the blood smears) and Vincent's angina, respectively.

FUNGI

Overview

Fungi are roughly divided into two morphologic types: yeasts and molds. There is also a dimorphic type that changes from a yeast to a mold, and vice versa, depending on temperature. The dimorphs are the type most likely to cause systemic disease in the immunocompetent host. The dimorphic fungi are also more limited in environment. The infecting form of fungi is usually spores (molds) which convert to yeasts in a moist environment at body temperature. The Deuteromycetes are a class of fungus that contains the yeasts *Candida* and *Cryptococcus*, the molds which cause skin and nail disease (dermatophytes), and the dimorphic fungi: *Histoplasma*, *Coccidioides*, and *Blastomyces*. *Mucor* is of the class Phycomycetes (nonseptate hyphae), and *Aspergillus* is of the genus Ascomycetes.

CANDIDA

Candida albicans should be considered as a cause of infection in immunosuppressed patients, patients on antibiotics or doing poorly despite antibiotics, and patients with uncontrolled diabetes. It is also seen in patients with indwelling catheters. Diagnosis: on physical exam, disseminated candidiasis is indicated by finding a "cotton wool patch" on the retina. All orifices should be swabbed and any catheters removed. Send the swabs and catheter tips for KOH and C+S.

notes

Chronic mucocutaneous candidiasis is associated with a T cell problem in which the T cell does not recognize *Candida*. It usually starts at an age less than 2 years old. Patients present with a bad chronic oral and facial rash, alopecia, and occasionally, esophageal stricture. It is associated with polyglandular deficiency in which there can be hypoparathyroidism, Addison disease, DM, hypothyroidism, and/or vitiligo. These patients respond well to fluconazole. See pg 2-37 for Candida vaginitis.

Know that candidemia can result in three deadly syndromes:
1) Septic peripheral thrombophlebitis,
2) Septic thrombosis of the great central veins (especially with central venous catheters), and
3) Hepatosplenic candidiasis-this should be considered in recovering leukemia patients who present with fever and have negative cultures. CT scan shows focal areas of involvement of the liver.

All of these are treated by removing any infecting catheter and giving amphotericin B or fluconazole. In addition, any suppurative peripheral vein must be resected. Septic thrombosis of great central veins should be suspected if there is edema of the upper body and/or candidemia persisting > 2 days after removal of the catheter.

Treatment: even transient candidemia is now treated because of the increased possibility of secondary vertebral osteomyelitis, hepatic abscess, and endophthalmitis. Drugs used to treat candidemia are amphotericin B and fluconazole
- Amphotericin B: A total dose of 500 mg of amphotericin is suggested. Great vein thrombosis, endocarditis, and osteomyelitis require higher total doses of amphotericin B for cure (up to 1 gram).
- Fluconazole: the less severely ill can be given fluconazole 400 mg q day—initially given intravenously.

CRYPTOCOCCUS

Cryptococcus usually causes minimally symptomatic, self-limited infections. Patients may have a low grade fever, cough, and a pulmonary infiltrate—all which resolve. It is not associated with any particular geographical location. Although it is found in old pigeon droppings, most patients have no recollection of being in contact with any. Cryptococcal pneumonia may form cavitary lesions and peripheral "cannon ball" skin lesions.

Dissemination is more likely in T-cell deficient patients (AIDS, corticosteroid therapy, Hodgkin disease, ALL, diabetes, and those who are post-organ transplant). These patients are especially likely to get cryptococcal meningoencephalitis—the most common presentation of severe cryptococcus infection.

Presence of the organism is confirmed with a CSF cryptococcal antigen test or with a CSF India ink test, which is positive when you see the large "halo" due to the thick capsule around the organism.

Cryptococcal meningitis is treated with amphotericin B and 5-fluorocytosine. Less severely ill patients can be treated with fluconazole. A loading dose of 800 mg for several days followed by 400 mg daily is generally used.

COCCIDIOIDES HISTO, BLASTO

Coccidioides and *Histoplasma* are dimorphs which are also discussed in the Pulmonology section. Both usually cause few problems except in immunocompromised patients.

The spores of *Coccidioides immitis* are found in the soil of the arid southwest U.S. and northern Mexico (often called "Valley Fever"—think of San Joaquin Valley or Death Valley). Once inhaled, it converts to a yeast which, days to weeks later, causes a self-limited, flu-like illness with arthralgias, erythema multiforme, and/or erythema nodosum. It often has a sarcoid-like presentation. Disease often results in a pulmonary "coin lesion." In immunocompromised patients, the disease is usually more severe (see AIDS-related infections on pg 2-29). Think of this in a patient from Arizona with a sarcoid-like presentation! Fluconazole is the DOC for chronic coccidioidomycosis.

Histoplasma is confined to the Mississippi and Ohio river valleys and is especially found in bat and bird droppings. Do not confuse this with the "(death) valley fever" above. Histoplasmosis can present with interstitial pneumonia, palate ulcers, and splenomegaly. One third have anemia, neutropenia, or pancytopenia. The pneumonia and splenomegaly are similar to that seen in *C. psittaci* infection (pg 2-13). *Histoplasma* occasionally causes a cavitary pneumonia similar to that seen in TB. Acute pulmonary disease generally requires no therapy. Chronic or severe acute disease may be treated with itraconazole. Disseminated disease is usually treated with amphotericin B followed by itraconazole.

Blastomyces causes an illness similar to *Histo* and *Coccidio* above. It is seen in Arkansas and Wisconsin hunters and loggers. In addition, *Blasto* disseminates to the skin, causing crusted lesions. Bone lesions are commonly seen in blastomycosis. Treatment is with itraconazole.

DERMATOPHYTES

Dermatophytes are the skin and hair fungi. Ringworm (*Tinea corporis*) can be treated with topical clotrimazole or undecylenic acid. Then, if no success, itraconazole or terbinafine are the preferred oral agents. Never amphotericin.

SPOROTRICHOSIS

Sporotrichosis is caused by *Sporothrix schenckii*— a dimorphic fungus associated with plants. Gardeners tend to get it, often after being pricked by a thorn. Of the 4 types of clinical presentation, the cutaneous and the lymphangitic (nodules form on the skin over lymph channels) types are treated with ORAL potassium iodide or itraconazole, while the pulmonary and disseminated types are treated with amphotericin B or itraconazole. Sporotrichosis can be a chronic problem. The disseminated type is more common in immunodeficient gardeners! Warn those post-transplant rose gardeners! Remember that *Mycobacterium marinum* can cause similar lesions over lymphatic channels (see pg 2-38).

notes

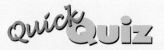

1) What type of fungal pneumonia can cause cavitary lesions and "cannon ball" skin lesions?

2) A patient presents on the examination with a central venous catheter infection due to *Candida albicans*. Do you have to remove the catheter?

3) What test must you do on the CSF of a 1 month post-transplant patient with signs of meningitis?

4) What is the treatment for sporotrichosis?

5) What dose the buzzphrase "diabetic with a black necrotic area in the paranasal sinuses" suggest?

6) What disease is suggested in an AIDS patient with multiple mass lesions of the brain?

7) How does cryptosporidiosis present in immunocompetent hosts? In immunocompromised?

MUCORMYCOSIS

Mucormycosis can be caused by *Mucor*, *Rhizopus*, and *Cunninghamella* organisms. Pulmonary mucormycosis affects immunocompromised patients, causing pulmonary infarcts. In diabetics, sinusitis is more common. Rhinocerebral mucormycosis starts as a black necrotic spot on the nose or paranasal sinuses and extends intracranially; it has a poor prognosis. Treat it with amphotericin B and debridement. Know that both *Aspergillus* and *Mucor* can cause a necrotizing, cavitating pneumonia.

PARASITES

PROTOZOA

Overview of Protozoa

There are two main types of parasites, Protozoa and Helminthic organisms. See Table 2-2

The protozoa are single celled and can replicate within the body so it only takes a small number of organisms to cause infection. Protozoa do NOT cause eosinophilia. The three TYPES OF PROTOZOA are:

- **I.** Sporozoa-*Toxoplasma*, *Cryptosporidia*, *Isospora*, *Pneumocystis* (although recent data supports this more as a FUNGUS!), *Plasmodium*, *Babesia*)
- **II.** Ameba
- **III.** Flagellates (*Giardia*, *Trichomonas*, *Trypanosoma*, *Leishmania*).

I. Sporozoa

Toxoplasma gondii

Toxoplasma gondii is the protozoa which causes toxoplasmosis. Cats are the definitive host as all the oocysts (infectious form) which eventually infect humans are shed in cat feces. It is common; 2/3 of adults have had it. Diagnosis is usually made by finding an elevated IgM antibody. There are 4 types of toxoplasmosis:

1) In the immunocompetent, it is most often asymptomatic, but may cause nontender lymphadenopathy, night sweats, and atypical lymphs. Self-limited.

2) It is serious in the immunocompetent only if acquired during pregnancy when it causes congenital toxoplasmosis (causing mental retardation and necrotizing chorioretinitis). The fetus is more likely to have a congenital infection if the disease is acquired later in pregnancy (15% 1st trimester; 70% last trimester but those infected later in pregnancy are usually asymptomatic).

3) Immunocompromised patients tend to get CNS infection and multiple mass lesions caused by a reactivation of a latent infection. AIDS patients remain on therapy for life. Tx: pyrimethamine and sulfadiazine.

4) Ocular toxoplasmosis causes retinal lesions that look like yellow-white cotton patches and also causes irregular scarring and pigmentation (disseminated candidiasis produces white cotton wool patches). Treatment consists of pyrimethamine and a sulfonamide (sulfadiazine or trisulfapyrimidine) for 3 weeks.

Table 2-2: Classification of Parasites		
PROTOZOA (do not replicate within the body) (no eosinophilia)	Sporozoa	*Toxoplasma, Cryptosporidium, Isospora belli, Plasmodium, Pneumocystis, Babesia*
	Ameba	*Entameba histolytica*
	Flagellates	*Giardia* - GI; *Trichomonas* - GU *Leishmania, Trypanosomes* - blood
HELMINTHS (do not replicate within the body) (+ eosinophilia)	Nemathelminthes (= nematodes) (= roundworms)	Pinworms, Hookworms, Whipworms (*Trichuris trichiura*), *Trichinella, Strongyloides*
	Platyhelminthes	Cestodes (tapeworms); Trematodes (flukes)

notes

Cryptosporidium

Cryptosporidium is a protozoan which causes infection especially in the immunocompromised, but also in the immunocompetent. The oocytes are passed in animal (including human) feces (vs. just cats in toxo). Symptoms in immunocompetent patients usually consist of a watery diarrhea which is self-limited, lasting 1-2 weeks. In the immunosuppressed, it can persist indefinitely and is refractory to medications—recent information shows that a combo of paromomycin + azithromycin may be helpful. Diagnose by acid-fast stains (small and round).

Isospora belli

Isospora belli is another acid-fast protozoa which causes a watery diarrhea in AIDS patients identical to Cryptosporidium. On the acid-fast stain, it is large and oval, whereas Cryptosporidium is small and round. Treat with TMP/SMX.

Cyclospora

Cyclospora is a newly described, acid fast intestinal protozoan parasite causing diarrhea in immunocompromised and immunocompetent patients. Clue: RASBERRIES from Guatemala! Systemic symptoms such as malaise, myalgia, low grade fever, and fatigue are commonly seen with *Cyclospora* infection. Treat with TMP/SMX.

Pneumocystis carinii is one of the most common causes of pneumonia in AIDS patients. It is covered in the Pulmonary section.

Malaria

Malaria [pg 16, #47-48]—*Plasmodium* is a protozoan which causes malaria. It affects the RBCs and is transmitted via the *Anopheles* mosquito. There are 4 types: *Plasmodium vivax, ovale, malariae,* and *falciparum.* Asplenic patients have more severe cases of malaria.

P. falciparum is the worst type of malaria. It is the cause of virtually all the fatal infections. It also has widespread chloroquine-resistance. Most cases of *P. falciparum* are acquired in mid-Africa. The blood smear in *P. falciparum* shows "banana gametophytes" and often you see more than one infected RBC on the slide, and even multiple parasitized RBCs.

This greatly contrasts with the other forms of malaria in which the parasitized RBCs are often hard to find. Finding a banana gametophyte on the peripheral blood smear is diagnostic of *P. falciparum.* Even though *P. falciparum* causes the highest levels of parasitemia, the schizonts are not seen on peripheral smear. If you see schizonts, the patient has one of the other types.

The Duffy RBC antigen is the site of attachment for *P. vivax.* Any type of malaria can cause nephritis from immune complex deposition but *P. malariae* is most commonly associated with nephrotic syndrome. Antibody production causes a decrease in parasitemia, but not in the number of intracellular parasites!

Treatment (see Table 2-3): Chloroquine is used for infections of *Plasmodium vivax, P. ovale,* and *P. malariae.* Primaquine is adjunctive medication for infections with *P. vivax* and *P. ovale* to eradicate hypnozoites in the liver. Hypnozoites are the malarial forms responsible for relapse. Chloroquine sensitive *P. falciparum* is treated with chloroquine, of course. If the *P. falciparum* is likely to be chloroquine-resistant, give quinine sulfate/gluconate, et. al., as shown in Table 2-3. Another option is mefloquine (Lariam®). Mefloquine is effective against chloroquine-resistant, and even Fansidar-resistant, *P. falciparum.* It is also effective against the chloroquine-sensitive plasmodia.

Remember, the use of pyrimethamine/sulfadoxine (Fansidar®) is rarely associated with the risk of severe Stevens-Johnson syndrome (which is due to the sulfa)! Also remember, primaquine induces hemolytic anemia in G-6-PD deficient persons, so you must screen for G-6-PD deficiency before prescribing it.

For malaria prophylaxis, chloroquine is usually used if no chloroquine-resistant Falciparum malaria is present in the

Table 2-3: Prophylaxis and Treatment of Malaria		
TYPE OF MALARIA	TREATMENT	PROPHYLAXIS
Nonfalciparum malaria	Chloroquine and primaquine.	Chloroquine 500mg (300 mg base) weekly. Give daily in endemic areas.
P. falciparum Chloroquine sensitive	Chloroquine Malarone	
P. falciparum Chloroquine resistant Not very ill.	Quinine sulfate p.o. plus either Fansidar, doxycycline, or clindamycin. or Mefloquine 15-25mg/kg; 1,250 mg max - single oral dose. or Malarone: 4 po qd daily x 3 days	Mefloquine: one dose weekly including 1 wk before and 4 wks after Malarone: one dose daily including 1-2 days before and 7d after
P. falciparum Chloroquine resistant Very ill.	IV quinidine gluconate +/- IV clindamycin. When better, change to p.o. quinine and clindamycin.	

notes

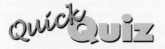

area in question. It should be started 1 to 2 weeks before arrival to the endemic area and be continued 4-6 weeks after leaving the area. Mefloquine is used for prophylaxis in chloroquine-resistant areas. Primaquine can be given the last 2 weeks of a prophylaxis period with either chloroquine or mefloquine after travel to areas where there is *P. vivax* or *P. ovale*. Know that the main causes of malaria in the U.S. are either not taking prophylaxis or stopping prophylaxis too soon after returning from travels to endemic areas!

Malarone, a fixed combination of atovaquone and proguanil, has recently been approved for the prophylaxis and treatment of uncomplicated *P. falciparum* malaria. For prophylaxis, the advantage is that it can be started just prior to leaving and stopped soon after return and has fewer side effects while the disadvantage is that it must be taken daily.

Babesia

Babesia microti is an intra-RBC protozoan parasite which causes babesiosis. This disease is a febrile hemolytic anemia seen especially in debilitated elderly patients and asplenic patients. The organism is transmitted via the *Ixodes* tick from rodents (as is the spirochete *Borrelia*, which causes Lyme disease). It is mostly seen in the Northeast US—usually in summer or early autumn.

Symptoms, which may persist for months, include fever, profuse sweats, myalgias, and shaking chills. Hemoglobinuria is a predominate sign. Patients often are emotionally labile. Because of the symptoms and the parasitized RBCs, it may be misdiagnosed as malaria.

B. microti is distinguished from *Plasmodium* by the classic intra-RBC tetrad appearing as a "Maltese Cross" but which more often looks more like four dots in a square shape (the malaria parasites have a ring form).

Mild babesiosis infections are usually self-limited. Treat moderate infections with clindamycin plus quinine or atovaquone plus azithromycin. If severe, do an exchange transfusion, then give antibiotics. Again, asplenic patients have more severe disease.

II. AMEBIASIS

Human amebiasis is caused by the protozoa *Entamoeba histolytica* [pg 16, #46]. Transmission is fecal-oral and can be food or water-borne. In the U.S., the usual population groups in which it is found are the institutionalized, immigrants, and homosexual men. For intestinal disease the diagnosis is made by examining the stool. However, the aspirate of an amebic liver abscess often shows no ameba or PMNs—DX: serology!

Metronidazole is the treatment of choice—even large amebic abscesses respond very quickly.

III. FLAGELLATES

The flagellates: *Giardia lamblia, Trichomonas vaginalis, Trypanosoma, Leishmania.*

Giardia lamblia

Giardia infections are found in campers, travelers, children in day-care, homosexuals, and in patients with IgA deficiency and/or hypogammaglobulinemia. It infects the duodenum. (Remember that *Shigella* is also found among day-care kids and homosexuals). 75% of infected persons are asymptomatic. Acute symptoms include a watery, smelly diarrhea and flatulence. Chronic giardiasis causes flatulence, sulfuric belching, and soft stools. Diagnose with microscopic examination of fresh stool samples x 3 or Giardia antigen test on one stool. For chronic giardiasis, a string test may be required: have the patient swallow a capsule on a string, leave it for several hours, and then retrieve it and check for trophozoites—this is rarely done today. Treat with metronidazole or quinacrine.

Trichomonas vaginalis

Trichomonas vaginalis causes an STD. Treat with metronidazole. More under Vaginitis, pg 2-37.

Trypanosomiasis

Trypanosomiasis is caused by *Trypanosoma*. There are 2 main types. The African disease is sleeping sickness. It is caused by *Trypanosoma brucei* and is transmitted via the tsetse fly. The American illness, Chagas' disease, is caused by *T. cruzi*; it is found in South America and Mexico. Usually it is self limited, but the chronic form can cause problems with the heart (from heart block to CHF), GI system (especially achalasia, megaesophagus, and megacolon as discussed in GI section), and occasionally the CNS.

Leishmaniasis

Leishmaniasis is caused by any of the following 4 species of the *Leishmania* protozoa: *L. donovani, L. tropica, L. mexicana,* and *L. braziliensis. L. donovani* is spread by a sand fly

notes

and causes visceral leishmaniasis, also called kala-azar. These patients get GI symptoms, hepatomegaly, and sometimes huge splenomegaly. The other species cause cutaneous and mucocutaneous forms of the disease.

Sodium stibogluconate (pentavalent antimony) is the treatment of choice—available from the CDC. Amphotericin B and itraconazole have been used with some success for cutaneous leishmaniasis.

HELMINTHIC ORGANISMS

Overview

The HELMINTHIC ORGANISMS are the other major type of parasite (remember: 1) Protozoa and 2) Helminthic organisms). They are multicellular worms that, in general, do not replicate in the body—and they DO cause eosinophilia. The two types of helminthic organisms are:
1) Nemathelminthes, the nematodes or roundworms which include pinworms, hookworms, whipworms (*Trichuris trichiura*), *Trichinella,* and *Strongyloides* and
2) Platyhelminthes, which include cestodes (tapeworms) and trematodes (flukes).

Nematodes (roundworm)

Nematodes are the roundworms. We will mention 8 types:
1) Roundworm (*Ascaris lumbricoides*)
2) Pinworm (*Enterobius*, causes rectal itching),
3) Hookworm (e.g., *Necator americanus*, causes anemia, weakness and fatigue, also can cause cutaneous larva migrans) [pg 17, #49]
4) Whipworm (Trichiura)
5) *Trichinella spiralis* larvae, which are usually found in pork (but also found in many carnivores), cause trichinosis. Although only ~50 cases per year are diagnosed in the U.S., the overall frequency of infection found on autopsy is ~4%!
6) *Wuchereria bancrofti* is transmitted by the mosquito. It is one of the causes of lymphatic filariasis (lymphatic blockage) and 2° elephantiasis! It may take thousands of bites by infected mosquitoes to inoculate enough of the organism to cause this (remember, with the exception of *Strongyloides*, helminthic organisms do not multiply in the human body). Diagnose by presence of microfilariae in the blood.
7) *Strongyloides stercoralis* is the least common of the nematodes in the U.S. but is very common in South America and Southeast Asia. Highly endemic areas exist in Southeast Asia and South America, where up to 60% of the population is infected. In the US, studies found infection rates of 3% among Kentucky school children and 6% at the Tennessee VA hospital.

It is (virtually) the only helminthic organism that replicates in the body. With this autoinfection, the infection can persist for decades (*Strong*!).

Symptoms are usually GI but there can be pulmonary symptoms during the infective part of the larvae's life cycle. Eosinophilia usually is present.

In immunosuppressed patients, potentially fatal disseminated strongyloidiasis may occur—presenting with abdominal pain and distension, neuro and pulmonary symptoms, and shock.

Diagnose with serial stool samples. Treat with ivermectin or thiabendazole.

8) *Toxocara canis* (and sometimes *Toxocara cati*) cause visceral larva migrans. The normal host for *Toxocara canis* is dogs and it is transmitted to humans by ingesting soil contaminated with dog excreta. In humans, the larvae do not develop into adult worms but rather migrate through the host tissue—eliciting eosinophilia. In the U.S., Toxocara seropositivity is 20% in kindergarten children and 2% in the general population. Treatment is with albendazole or mebendazole.

Platyhelminthes (cestodes and trematodes)

Platyhelminthes include cestodes (tapeworms) and trematodes (flukes).

Cestodes are the flatworms (tapeworms). The pork tapeworm, *Taenia solium*, has two clinical entities:
1) If the cysticerci are ingested, taeniasis develops (a tapeworm grows in the intestines).
2) If an egg-contaminated food is ingested (from animal or human feces), the patient will develop CYSTICERCOSIS. In this, the eggs hatch and the oncospheres go into the blood and, most significantly, cause cysticerci in the CNS and eyes. These cysts do nothing until the organism dies. In the brain (neurocysticercosis), the resulting inflammation usually causes seizures as the first symptom. Especially consider cysticercosis in a patient with new onset seizures who is a Mexican immigrant or from a household with a Mexican immigrant.

Niclosamide is the usual treatment for all intestinal tapeworms. Albendazole (first choice) or praziquantel along with corticosteroids are used for neurocysticercosis. NOTE: IF OCULAR OR SPINAL CYSTS ARE PRESENT DO NOT TREAT—CAUSES IRREPARABLE DAMAGE.

Trematodes are the flukes.
1) *Clonorchis sinensis* is the Chinese liver fluke. It is endemic in the Far East; infection is caused by eating raw fish and it is often associated with biliary obstruction.
2) *Schistosoma haematobium* infects the bladder causing urinary symptoms.
3) *Schistosoma mansoni* is a fluke found in Africa, Middle East, and South America while
4) *Schistosoma japonicum* is found in Asia.

Schistosoma causes acute schistosomiasis (Katayama fever [pg 17, #50]) about 2 months after inoculation. This infection presents with fever, lymphadenopathy, diarrhea (DDX: travelers' diarrhea), hepatosplenomegaly, and marked eosinophilia. The most serious complication of schistosomiasis is cirrhosis with esophageal varices. Schistosomiasis does not cause the other stigmata seen with alcoholic cirrhosis (spiders, gynecomastia, or ascites).

Diagnosis is made by finding the eggs in the stool.

Praziquantel, given for one day!, is the drug of choice for any *Schistosoma* and most other fluke infections.

notes

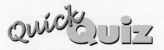

Quick Quiz

1) A veteran of World War II develops severe pulmonary and GI problems after starting chemotherapy. What is the most likely worm to do this?

2) An immigrant from Mexico presents with new-onset seizures. Which flatworm is a possible etiology for their seizure? What is the treatment? When do you *not* treat.

3) For which viruses is a Tzanck smear effective as a diagnostic tool? What does it show when positive for this virus?

4) Can Herpes be spread without lesions being present?

VIRUSES

HSV

Herpes Simplex Virus (HSV): A DNA virus.

HSV-1 causes orofacial infections in about 40% of the population [pg 6, #16]. In the primary infection, the vesicular lesions and ulcers are usually localized to the oral mucosa, lips, and surrounding skin, whereas in recurrent infections, ulcers are usually on the outer lip. Tzanck test is done by scraping down to the bottom cellular layer of a vesicle, placing the material on a slide, and then staining with either Giemsa or Wright—in herpes simplex and varicella (including zoster) it will show multinucleated giant cells. It is possible to autoinoculate the virus, so the infection can be spread from the lips (or other areas) to the eyes of a patient. Recurrent HSV-1 eye infection resulting in a keratitis is the most common infectious cause of blindness in industrialized nations [pg 6, #18].

HSV-2 causes "genital herpes" [pg 6, #17]. Actually it causes about 75% of HSV genital infections—the rest are due to Type 1. Note that the prevalence of HSV-2 is 25% and, of those, only 25% have symptoms!! In 10% of patients, the initial occurrence of HSV-2 is associated with only a herpetic exudative pharyngitis. New data suggests many HSV infections are spread by asymptomatic shedding of virus.

Most cases of neonatal HSV are from intrapartum contact, so a C-section is recommended if the mother has symptoms or signs of genital herpes or its prodrome at the time of delivery. The risk for transmission to the neonate is high (30-50%) among women who get their 1st episode of genital herpes near the time of delivery and is low (<1%) among women with a history of recurrent herpes. HSV reactivates in 2/3 of seropositive transplant patients within 6 weeks of transplant.

> **HERPES VIRUSES**
>
> The herpes viruses are double stranded DNA viruses which include the herpes simplex viruses (HSV-I and HSV-2), CMV, Epstein-Barr, and varicella-zoster viruses.

HSV causes the highest number of deaths due to encephalitis in adults (the most commonly **identified** etiologies are due to arboviruses but the majority of encephalitis cases today are still not identified). Patients with herpes encephalitis usually present with constitutional symptoms and altered mental status and may have focal neurologic signs. Because it has a predilection for the temporal lobe, patients may have temporal lobe seizure symptoms (abnormal behavior, smells burning rubber). More than 60% are left with neurologic sequelae! The EEG and MRI are the tests most sensitive for diagnosis.

HSV is one of the many causes of erythema multiforme (See Dermatology section).

Treatment of HSV: acyclovir is used for all the types of herpes infections. It is given IV in the immunosuppressed patients (but careful, may cause acute renal insufficiency!). It, or one of its analogs (famciclovir, valacyclovir), is given orally for genital herpes. Acyclovir (or famciclovir, or valacyclovir) can also be given chronically to suppress infection, or as a treatment for acute recurrence. Foscarnet is used to treat HSV resistant to acyclovir; ganciclovir is not used.

Varicella-zoster virus (VZV; DNA) causes chickenpox and herpes zoster (shingles). Symptoms of chickenpox are usually mild in children but they may be severe in adolescents and adults and especially pregnant women [pg 7, #19]; pneumonia is more likely to occur in these older patients. In the mother, besides increased severity and pneumonia, if she is infected between 8 and 20 weeks, birth defects are more likely.

Current recommendation is for pregnant patients exposed to chicken pox to receive zoster immune globulin (ZIG or VZIG) within 4 days of exposure. If over 4 days, it does no good. Do not give varicella virus vaccine (Varivax®) to pregnant patients as it is a live vaccine.

Most authorities recommending treating adults/adolescents with oral acyclovir 800 mg qid x 5 days if they present within the first 24 hours of the exanthem. An immunocompromised patient should receive IV acyclovir (toxicity: acute renal insufficiency!)

Herpes zoster (shingles) is caused by reactivation of the *Varicella-zoster* virus [pg 7, #20-21]. A Tzanck smear will show multinucleated giant cells which are pathognomonic for herpes viruses. Post-herpetic neuralgia is more likely with increasing age. Shingles recurs in less than 5% of nonimmunosuppressed patients.

Prednisone, previously used with acyclovir, prolongs the course of Herpes zoster in immunosuppressed patients. Immunosuppressed patients often get severe cases of shingles. Although it was previously thought that prednisone decreases the incidence of post-herpetic neuralgia in the immunocompetent, well designed studies have shown no benefit.

High dose oral acyclovir alone can be used to treat zoster; although it shortens the course of acute illness a little, it does not decrease the incidence of post-herpetic neuralgia. Only famciclovir and valacyclovir are shown to decrease the incidence of post-herpetic neuralgia. Valacyclovir is an L-valyl ester of acyclovir, has 3-5x greater bioavailability than acyclovir, and is almost completely converted to acyclovir after oral administration. For pain control tricyclics, gabapentin, and lidocaine patches have some efficacy. Narcotics are effective and UNDERUSED in this instance! Amitriptyline (Elavil®) may be helpful for treatment of post-herpetic neuralgia.

If a patient presents with back pain and you think it is a Herpes zoster prodrome, what should you do? Answer: nothing except follow closely. The acyclovir or its analogs is not started until vesicles are seen.

CMV

Cytomegalovirus (CMV) is a DNA virus. CMV infection is usually asymptomatic and fairly common. One half of the population has anti-CMV antibodies by the age of 35. CMV is a very common infection in patients with decreased cellular immunity (post-transplant and AIDS). 75% of seronegative transplant recipients get CMV if the donor is seropositive. With a post-transplant systemic CMV infection, the patient can have concurrent "-itises" which may include encephalitis, hepatitis, retinitis, colitis, and adrenalitis (causing adrenal insufficiency); these are especially common and more severe if the recipient is seronegative prior to the transplant.

CMV is the usual cause of eye problems in AIDS patients with low CD4 count. CMV can cause chorioretinitis, pneumonitis, esophagitis, and colitis. The CMV retinitis is distinctive; it has both retinal blanching and hemorrhage. Diagnosis is confirmed if CMV is cultured from the buffy coat smear. CMV pneumonitis in transplant patients is diagnosed by finding inclusion bodies on the biopsy specimen.

CMV chorioretinitis (usually in AIDS patients) is treated with ganciclovir (DHPG), foscarnet or combination of both. Also intraocular ganciclovir release devices with oral ganciclovir have been effective. Cidofovir is also approved. However, all of these agents only have a suppressive effect and must be given until T-lymphocyte count increases to > 200.

Major toxicities of ganciclovir include granulocytopenia (30%!!) and low platelets. ZDV (pg 2-25) also causes granulocytopenia and patients occasionally cannot tolerate both. The major toxicity of foscarnet is reversible renal failure; it also causes hypocalcemia, hypomagnesemia, and hyperphosphatemia (patients may present with seizures). Because they are only suppressive, these drugs do not cure the symptoms and once stopped, the disease resumes.

EBV

Epstein-Barr Virus (DNA) causes infectious mononucleosis [pg 8, #22-23]. Incubation period is 1-2 months. Most (>90%) patients have pharyngitis or tonsillitis, fever, lymphadenopathy, and abnormal liver function. Lymphocytosis is common with >10% atypical lymphocytes: enlarged with abundant cytoplasm, vacuoles, and indentations of the cell membrane. Half have splenomegaly. Most develop a macular rash if given ampicillin. Heterophil antibody titers (monospot) decrease within 6 months, but the EB IgG antibodies are present for years. The atypical lymphs are T cells. Recurrence is unusual but possible—usually with high titers of antibody to EB antigen (>1:5000).

EBV causes hairy leukoplakia; this mucocutaneous lesion may be seen as an early manifestation of HIV disease [pg 2, #5]. High dose acyclovir may offer some benefit in treatment of oral hairy leukoplakia. Chronic fatigue has no proven association with EB virus. The EBV is also associated with nasopharyngeal carcinoma and Burkitt's lymphoma.

A patient with mononucleosis symptoms who is heterophil-negative usually has CMV.

RUBELLA

Rubella is "German measles" (ss RNA virus) [pg 4, #11]. If it is acquired by a pregnant patient in the first trimester, there is a 50% chance that the baby will have congenital defects. It is diagnosed by the hemagglutination inhibition test. If this test is negative in a newly exposed pregnant patient, it should be repeated in 3 weeks (after incubation period) before any decisions are made. If it is then positive, the patient should be offered the option of a therapeutic abortion. Immune globulin does not prevent the infection, but it may give some fetal protection in the patient who refuses therapeutic abortion.

RUBEOLA

Rubeola is "measles" [pg 4, #12]. Symptoms start ~10 days after the initial exposure. Symptoms at the onset: the "3 Cs": cough, coryza, and conjunctivitis (with photophobia). They also have malaise and fever. Koplik's spots (whitish spots on an erythematous base) appear on the buccal mucosa 2-3 days before the onset of the skin rash. The skin rash starts at the hairline and spreads downward. It lasts ~5 days and then resolves, also from the hairline downward. Again: 3 Cs, Koplik spots, rash.

RETROVIRUS

Retroviruses—RNA viruses. HTLV-1 causes T-cell leukemia. HTLV-2 causes a rare T-cell variant of hairy cell leukemia. HIV, previously called HTLV-3, causes AIDS. HIV-2, found in W. Africa and parts of the United States, is virus which causes an illness indistinguishable from AIDS (both HIV I and II are now picked up by ELISA). More on HIV later.

RESPIRATORY VIRUSES

• Rhinoviruses are a common cause of URI in adults—usually during the autumn.

• Respiratory syncytial virus (RSV) infections occur yearly, during the autumn and winter. RSV infections are more severe in the infant, occasionally resulting in pneumonia. Only

notes

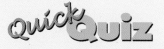

1% of affected infants are hospitalized. Diagnose RSV by doing an ELISA test on nasal secretions.

• Influenza is still a major cause of death, especially if the patient is > 55 years old with COPD. Vaccination decreases mortality by 1/3!

There are three types of influenza viruses: Influenza A, B, and C. A&B cause the yearly epidemics of respiratory illnesses. Influenza C causes very mild if any symptoms.

Treatment of influenza:

Amantadine and rimantadine are not only protective against infection with influenza A (A-A) but they also decrease the severity of infection if given within 24 hours of onset of symptoms. Amantadine/rimantadine dosage must be adjusted for any renal impairment.

Oseltamivir (Tamiflu®—oral) and zanamivir (Relenza®— powder for inhalation) are the first of the neuraminidase inhibitors, a newer class of treatment for influenza A & B (FDA approved 1999). If given within 48 hours of onset of symptoms, it decreases duration by 30%. If given within 12 hours it decreases duration by 50%. It also prevents clinical disease in over 90% of household contacts.

When an influenza A epidemic threatens an unimmunized nursing home, who should get amantadine or rimantadine? Answer: the entire population of the nursing home...and give the influenza vaccine to all who have not yet been vaccinated for that season.

Vaccinations are covered in the General Internal Medicine section.

POLIO

Polio—90% is self limited. Its onset is characterized by an aseptic meningitis and an asymmetric, flaccid paralysis without reflexes. It is essentially eliminated in the western hemisphere and developed countries worldwide. More in the Neurology section.

RABIES

Rabies [pg 5, #14]—especially found in bats, raccoons, skunks, and foxes. Not squirrels. If the animal is not available for rabies evaluation and if the last vaccine was given > 6 years ago, give the vaccine and rabies immune globulin. Prophylaxis is indicated for cave explorers and veterinarians but not hunters, mailmen etc.

MUMPS

Mumps (RNA [pg 5, #13]) occurs most commonly in winter and early spring. Although it often is asymptomatic, it can present with uni- or bilateral parotitis, aseptic meningitis, and/or encephalitis. 15-20% of post-pubertal males with mumps get an epididymo-orchitis which is usually unilateral. Post infection sterility is a rare occurrence. To differentiate between mumps and bacterial parotitis, just check a gram stain of the parotid secretions. There are many WBCs and organisms in bacterial parotitis and none in mumps.

Note: another cause of enlarged parotid glands is frequent vomiting. Always consider bulimia in an adult with parotid gland enlargement.

PARVOVIRUS

Parvovirus is a small DNA virus. One parvovirus, B19, causes various disorders ranging from erythema infectiosum ("Fifth disease") to arthralgias/arthritis to aplastic anemia. Erythema infectiosum is a mildly contagious, self-limited infection which causes a rash and arthritis. The facial component of the rash causes a "slapped cheek" appearance [pg 5, #15]. This rash is much more common in children and the arthritis is more common in adults. It is in patients with chronic hemolytic anemias or AIDS that it can cause aplastic anemia. In these, the bone marrow shows characteristic "giant pronormoblasts".

HANTAVIRUS

Hantavirus. There is a hantavirus-associated disease called Hantavirus Pulmonary Syndrome (HPS) which starts with severe myalgias, fever, headache, and cough and quickly progresses to ARDS and death. More than 50% die. The primary reservoir in the U.S. is the deer mouse. On the eastern coast and in the southeast, the cotton rat is the main reservoir. The infection occurs when the excreta or saliva are inhaled.

notes

Transfer of the virus can also occur through the broken skin. No person-to-person transfer is known to occur.

Symptoms:

Early = constitutional symptoms in all. About half have N/V, diarrhea, and abdominal pain.

Late: 4-10 days later = coughing and shortness of breath as ARDS develops.

NO RASH.

DENGUE FEVER

Dengue fever, dengue hemorrhagic fever, and dengue shock syndrome are cause by 4 serotypes of the Flavivirus. It is a tropical disease which uses humans and the day-biting *Aedes* mosquitos (*Anopheles* carry malaria) in its life-cycle. Dengue fever has had a resurgence the last 10 years in South America and Mexico and a few cases in South Texas. No vaccine is available yet (under development).

Symptoms are rapid onset of high fever, severe myalgias and arthralgias ("break-bone fever"), and severe headaches with N/V followed by a macular red rash which covers most of the body. A second rash that looks more like measles occurs later along with a recurrence of fever ("saddleback fever"—up down up).

Suspect this in a traveler with these symptoms who has returned from tropical latitudes (including the Caribbean and Mexico). Treatment is supportive.

SLOW VIRUSES

Overview

There are 2 classes of slow viruses.

1) normal viruses such as papilloma (warts) and papovavirus (PML).

2) defective viruses such as the defective measles virus which causes subacute sclerosing panencephalitis

Papillomavirus

Papillomavirus causes warts. Genital warts are associated with an increased risk of cervical cancer [pg 18, #52] . Many variants. HPV #1,2, and 5 are common causes of plantar warts. HPV #6,11,16,18, and 31 are genital. HPV # 6 and 11 are the cause of the exophytic grossly visible genital warts but only HPV #16,18 and 31 are associated with cervical cancer (remember: higher numbers occur higher up on the body and are more cancer prone!). The HPV # 16, 18, and 31 which cause cervical cancer are usually subclinical! So do not jump to "cervical cancer!" when you see genital warts! All warts tend to recur.

Papovavirus

Papovavirus—reactivation in the immunosuppressed host results in Progressive Multifocal Leukoencephalopathy (PML) which is due to progressive demyelination of the white matter. PML, because it is multifocal, has varied presentations. Usually the patient suffers altered mental status followed by various focal motor/sensory defects. It is diagnosed by MRI.

SSPE

Subacute sclerosing panencephalitis (SSPE) is a rare form of encephalopathy thought to be due to a measles virus which had been changed, but not eradicated, by the immune reaction to the primary infection. Occurrence is 1/300,000 cases of measles. Patients usually had measles at an age of < 2 years and present with dementia, myoclonus, and new-onset seizures around the age of 10. Most die within several months of onset.

Prion Disease

Prions are proteinaceous infectious particles that lack nucleic acid and constitute a previously unknown means of transmitting disease. Previously, these diseases were thought to be caused by a "slow virus."

Prion diseases include Kuru, Creutzfeldt-Jakob disease (CJD), variant of CJD (vCJD), Gerstmann-Straussler-Schinker (GSS) syndrome, fatal familial insomnia. In animals: scrapie and mad cow disease (= bovine spongiform encephalopathy, = vCJD when transmitted to humans).

Human prion diseases can be sporadic (CJD), infectious (vCJD, kuru, rare cases of CJD), or genetic (GSS syndrome, familial CJD, fatal familial insomnia).

Kuru is found in New Guinea and is associated with cannibalism and is thought to be transmitted by ingestion of raw human brain tissue. It has an incubation period of up to 30 years. No new cases since ritual cannibalism has stopped.

Creutzfeldt-Jakob disease (CJD) is the most common prion disease. It is almost always sporadic but about 5% are infectious (e.g., corneal transplants, cadaveric human growth hormone), and very few are genetic. Its incubation period is about 18 months. Patients with CJD get myoclonus and severe dementia. Neurologic symptoms predominate. They generally die within 5 months! There is no effective therapy for either Kuru or CJD. The EEG is diagnostic.

A new variant of CJD (vCJD), probably transmitted from beef with bovine spongiform encephalopathy (mad cow disease), has been contracted by about 60 people in several European countries. No U.S. cases of vCJD have been reported. These patients have early-on psychiatric symptoms and late-appearing neurologic symptoms (about 6 months, ataxia). Once neurologic symptoms appear, progression to death is rapid. Test: Look for a young adult from England with progressive psychiatric symptoms and ataxia.

HIV and AIDS

OVERVIEW

Changes in the treatment and management of HIV infection is evolving rapidly. The following covers the basics—not the cutting edge.

notes

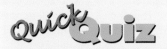

1) What viruses cause "break bone fever"? In what group of patients and with what symptoms would you consider this diagnosis?

2) What types of genital warts are cancer prone?

3) What encephalitis is associated with early childhood measles?

4) Which prion disease is associated with progressive dementia and excessive startle response?

5) On the Boards, what diagnosis should you consider in a young adult from England who presents with worsening psychiatric problems and dementia?

6) What is the best laboratory test to order to determine evidence of acute HIV infection?

7) Which common anti-HIV medication causes bone marrow suppression?

The virus particle:

The HIV virus is composed of a dense single-strand RNA core surrounded by a lipoprotein envelope. The RNA contains reverse transcriptase, which allows the RNA to be transcribed into DNA, which is then assimilated into the host's genome. The cell then becomes an HIV-producing machine.

The structure in the lipoprotein envelope which allows the HIV to attach to the CD4 cell is named gp120. As opposed to influenza, the envelope on HIV is very unstable and therefore it is much more difficult to make a vaccine against it.

HIV gp120 envelope glycoprotein binds to the CD4 receptors and coreceptors on the helper T cells, macrophages, and monocytes. The virus fuses with the cell and the viral core material enters the cell. Immune dysfunction results from the ongoing destruction of CD4 lymphocytes as will be more fully described under "Summary of Important Advances." The CD4 cells are the major regulator cells in the body. They can suppress the B lymphocytes, and regulate the CD8/suppressor cells.

With the decrease in CD4+ counts, B-cells become deregulated and are no longer suppressed, causing a polyclonal increase in total serum immunoglobulins even though overall antibody function is decreased! For this reason, infectious diseases in AIDS patients not only include the cell-mediated infections (PCP, viruses, *mycobacteria*, fungal) but also those seen with humoral deficiency (pneumococcus, meningococcus, *H. influenzae*, and *Giardia*).

The glial cells of the CNS may be directly affected by HIV, causing atrophy and dementia. The GI epithelium may be directly infected, causing a wasting enteropathy with diarrhea. Marrow progenitor cell infection may be the cause of anemia and thrombocytopenia.

Prevalence and transmission: HIV is positive among 50% of IV drug users and 50% of gays seeking treatment for STDs. Prevalence is < 1% in heterosexuals in the U.S., but in central Africa heterosexual transmission is the primary route! It has been transmitted by a dentist. Percentages of patients with AIDS: homosexuals (56%), IV drug users (24%), IV drug user & homosexual (5%), heterosexual contact (6%), hemophiliacs (1%), transfusion associated (2%).

HIV exposure is diagnosed by demonstrating the presence of antibody to the virus by means of the ELISA test which is 99% sensitive and 90% specific. Positive responders are confirmed by the Western blot. Antibody to HIV is usually detectable 2-3 months after inoculation although there can be a window up to 6 months! The earliest detectable sign of infection is a positive HIV PCR DNA.

There are several tests which measure HIV RNA by amplifying the RNA by oligonucleotide hybridization or enzymatic methods. These tests accurately determine viral load. They are discussed further below.

TREATMENT OF HIV INFECTION

Note

Treatment of HIV infection: Adherence is a key determinant in the degree and duration of viral suppression! AIDS: Note that it is extremely important to actively involve the patient in the treatment decision-making process. Decisions regarding initiation or changes in antiretroviral therapy should be guided by monitoring plasma HIV RNA (viral load) and CD4 T cell counts in addition to the patient's clinical condition. First we will review the four major classes of anti-HIV drugs and then treatment protocols.

Drug acronyms:

NRTI = Nucleoside Reverse Transcriptase Inhibitor
Nucleotide RTI = Nucleotide Reverse Transcriptase Inhibitor
NNRTI = NonNucleoside Reverse Transcriptase Inhibitor
PI = Protease Inhibitors

Nucleoside Reverse Transcriptase Inhibitors

I. Nucleoside Reverse Transcriptase Inhibitors (ZDV, ddI, ddC, d4T, 3TC, and abacavir—NRTI). These drugs inhibit the replication of HIV by interfering with the reverse transcriptase enzyme. These are all analogs of normally occurring nucleic acid bases.

Zidovudine (ZDV) = Azidothymidine (previously called AZT) = Retrovir® This is the oldest of the antiretroviral drugs but still remains very useful. It is well tolerated at currently used doses, but causes bone marrow suppression (anemia, granulocytopenia) and myopathy. A macrocytosis (elevated MCV) always occurs but has no clinical consequence. ZDV does not usually cause problems for the kidneys or lungs and does not cause pancreatitis.

As with all antiretroviral drugs, combination therapy is preferred and is the standard of care. ZDV is used in combination with 3TC, ddI, and ddC as well as protease inhibitors. Some studies have suggested antagonism between ZDV and d4T. The effectiveness of ZDV decreases over time due to development of resistance.

notes

ZDV should be given to HIV + pregnant patients because ZDV decreases transmission of the HIV virus to the fetus by 25-35%!

Because ganciclovir and ZDV have overlapping bone marrow toxicities, in an AIDS patient with CMV retinitis and on ZDV and ganciclovir, Filgrastim® (G-CSF) can be given to support the WBC. Sometimes it is necessary to stop the ganciclovir and use foscarnet.

ddI (didanosine, Videx®) is useful in combination regimens—with ZDV, d4T, and protease inhibitors. Viral resistance develops more slowly than with other reverse transcriptase inhibitors. A newer enteric coated tablet has replaced the regular preparation with elimination of the GI side-effects of diarrhea and cramping and hence much better patient tolerance.
The most severe side effects are pancreatitis, which can be life threatening, and peripheral neuropathy. There is no bone marrow toxicity.

ddC (zalcitabine, Hivid®) can be used as part of a combination regimen (the combination with ZDV is best studied). It is very easy to take and the only significant side effect is stomatitis and neuropathy and less commonly pancreatitis. Since the availability of newer drugs, ddC is rarely used.

d4T (stavudine, Zerit®) has emerged a very useful drug as it is very well tolerated over long periods of time with little toxicity. Well studied combinations include ddI/d4T and d4T/3TC with or without protease inhibitors. Recent data has implicated d4T in lipodystrophy and mitochondrial toxicity syndromes. Also d4T should not be used in combination with ddI in pregnant women—fatal lactic acidosis!
Side effects: especially pancreatitis and peripheral neuropathy.

3TC (lamivudine, Epivir®) is a very effective drug in combination therapy. Combinations with ZDV and d4T are often used. The drug is well tolerated.
Side effects are rare.

Abacavir (Ziagen®) is very effective in combination therapy.
Side effects: The most serious reaction is a hypersensitivity reaction which usually occurs within 4 weeks. The reaction consists of a generalized rash and/or a flu-like illness with fever, chills, N/V, myalgias, cough, and shortness of breath. Any patient that develops this reaction should be taken off abacavir and never take it again; reactions will continue to worsen and could even be fatal.

Combos: Currently there are 2 combo drugs: Combivir®=ZDV + 3TC and Trizivir®=ZDV + 3TC + Abacavir. Trizivir can be used as single therapy as it contains 3 NRTIs.

Nucleotide Reverse Transcriptase Inhibitor

Tenofovir (Viread ™) is a nucleotide RTI very similar to the above nucleoside analogues except that they are chemically preactivated and therefore require less biochemical processing than the nucleoside RTIs. Tenofovir has once-daily dosing and a good side-effect profile—mainly Asthenia/Headache/N/V/D/flatulence. It must be taken with a NRTI and at least one PI or NNRTI.

Non-nucleoside Reverse Transcriptase Inhibitors

II. Non-nucleoside reverse transcriptase inhibitors (NNRTI).
Nevirapine (Viramune®) is the first of this class of drugs. It is not useful as a single agent, but is useful as part of a regimen with nucleoside reverse transcriptase inhibitors and/or protease inhibitors. Rash, which can be severe, is the primary toxicity.
Efavirenz (Sustiva®); it is more potent than nevirapine. CNS toxicity is commonly seen. Efavirenz is teratogenic, so do not use around pregnancy. Other side effects include rash and "weird dreams".
Delavirdine (Rescriptor®) is less potent and therefore rarely used.

Protease Inhibitors

III. The HIV protease inhibitors—PI— (saquinavir, indinavir, ritonavir, nelfinavir, amprenavir, lopinavir) inhibit the HIV protease enzyme which is involved with processing the completed virus. They must either be used in combination with each other (e.g., saquinavir + ritonavir) OR with the just discussed NRTIs +/- NNRTI to prevent the emergence of resistance. Fat redistribution and lipid abnormalities (increased triglycerides and cholesterol) as well as new-onset diabetes have been recognized with the use of PIs. However in treating the lipid abnormalities do NOT use simvastatin or lovastatin with any of the PIs! Avoid other interactions: Rifampin, astemizole, cisapride and St. John's wort.
Saquinavir (Fortovase®) is highly effective, has minimum side effects, and is useful in combination protease inhibitor regimens.
Ritonavir (Norvir®) is a very potent drug but patient tolerability is poor due to side effects. The main side effects are N/V, flushing, distorted taste, and paresthesias. There are many drug interactions because of interference with the p450 enzyme system. Low dose ritonavir inhibits metabolism of and significantly boosts levels of indinavir, saquinavir, amprenavir, and the NNRTI efavirenz. Ritonavir is now usually used in low dose to boost the levels of other PIs and efavirenz.
Indinavir (Crixivan®) has side effects which include an asymptomatic hyperbilirubinemia and a high incidence of nephrolithiasis. The drug should be taken on an empty stomach with adequate hydration—although boosting with ritonavir eliminates the food requirement.
Nelfinavir (Viracept) is a PI with good potency. Well tolerated. Most common side effect is diarrhea. If resistance to nelfinavir develops, treatment with indinavir or amprenavir may be effective.
Amprenavir (Agenerase®) is a new PI with a resistance profile which is unique among protease inhibitors. 1% get serious

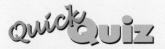

skin reactions, including Stevens-Johnson syndrome. GI side-effects are common.

Lopinavir/ritonavir (Kaletra®) is a coformulation of lopinavir and low-dose ritonavir. Lopinavir is available only in this coformulation. It is very potent and is well tolerated.

Key words

Key word/phrases to remember for side effects:
- ZDV: bone marrow suppression, myopathy
- The "D's" (ddI, ddC, and d4T): Pancreatitis and peripheral neuropathy.
- Abacavir (Ziagen®): Potentially fatal hypersensitivity reaction.
- Efavirenz (Sustiva®): teratogenic
- Indinavir (Crixivan®): kidney stones

Note for the medications above: *At least* know the Yellow-highlighted areas! That is what they are most likely to ask!

State of Treatment

I. Summary of important advances:

a) HIV RNA assays are available for accurately determining viral load. Prior to the availability of these assays, the HIV virus was thought to enter a prolonged latency period until the onset of symptoms. It turns out that there is continuous, high level replication from the onset of infection to death.

b) Viral load is a good, long-term predictor of outcome. After primary infection, the rate of virus replication and turnover equilibrates to a certain set point for each individual—resulting in a pretty much constant plasma viremia of 100 to 10^6 HIV RNA copies/mL. This set point may endure for months or years and it determines the rate of disease progression. Plasma viremia < 5 000 HIV RNA copies/mL is associated with near-normal CD4+ counts and minimal if any clinical progression of disease whereas viral loads > 30 000 HIV RNA copies/mL indicate a greatly increased risk of disease progression. Barring treatment, a single HIV RNA count

can establish a prognosis—similar to staging of certain malignancies.

Infected patients make up to 10^9 new HIV virions/day. The CD4+ lymphocytes, which are the principal cells targeted for reproducing HIV virions have a half-life of only 1.6 days after it is infected. High levels of viremia cause tremendous continuous CD4+ lymphocyte destruction—eventually causing decreased levels. Rather than using CD4+ cell level as a marker of disease activity (which is wrong—it is more an endpoint denoting prolonged disease activity), the present focus of treatment is to decrease viral load and thereby prevent or minimize the CD4+ cell destruction.

c) The HIV protease inhibitors decrease viral load—sometimes tremendously—for prolonged periods when used in combination therapy.

d) HIV therapy should always be combination therapy. Treat with PI(s) with NRTI(s) and/or NNRTI(s). Combinations of nucleoside analogues given to asymptomatic patients with early HIV disease and evidence of immunologic compromise (low CD4 counts) prolong survival and decrease AIDS-related problems. The combination therapy is superior to ZDV alone. Previously it was unknown if treating early in the course of the illness would improve outcome.

II. Pending questions:

a) Does the level of HIV RNA achieved by antiretroviral therapy have the same predictive value as that of untreated patients in the study? Studies suggest this is true. Each of the studies found a decreased risk of disease progression with treatment-induced decrease in HIV RNA level but did not address the actual levels.

b) How long-lasting is the effect of the protease inhibitor agents? HIV does mutate but the lower the viral load, the less the likelihood of resistance developing and the longer the regimen will be effective. Patients have been maintained without detectable virus for > 7 years.

c) What is the best combination of agents? Some guidelines (see below) but still vague...

d) When is the best time to start treatment? Some guidelines (see below) but still vague for asymptomatic patients…

III. The new treatment protocols are based on the above and:

- The probability that the decrease in viral load induced by combinations or HAART have the same predictive value as the studies mentioned in **I**b above.
- Determining CD4 and viral load are a key indicator for when to start therapy.
- Combination therapy is the standard of care and monotherapy should be used only in special circumstances.

Indications for Viral Load Testing:

1. Syndrome consistent with acute HIV
2. Initial evaluation of newly diagnosed HIV
3. Every 3-4 months for patients ON and NOT on therapy
4. 2-8 weeks after initiation of therapy

notes

5. Clinical event or substantial decline in CD4 Count

Indications for using drug-resistance assays

Resistance testing appears to be a useful tool in selecting active drugs when changing antiretroviral regimens in cases of virologic failure or suboptimal reduction of viral load. Currently two types of resistance testing are available—genotypic and phenotypic. These are expensive tests but are becoming more popular in determining optimal regimens. The genotypic test will detect specific genes in the individual patient's HIV virus known to confer resistance toward a specific antiretroviral drug. The phenotypic test determines if the gene is operating and if resistance is being expressed. Currently neither is recommended over the other and some centers prefer to test for both. This is sort of like a crude antibiogram for the HIV virus—if resistance is determined then you can switch from ineffective drugs.

When to initiate antiretroviral therapy:

• Definite:
  Symptomatic (AIDS or severe symptoms) start therapy no matter what the CD4 or Viral load
  Asymptomatic and CD4 is less than 200
• Almost Definite:
  Asymptomatic and CD4 is between 200 and 350
• Most recommend:
  Asymptomatic with CD4 above 350 and Viral Load is >55,000. (In untreated patients the 3-year risk for progression to AIDS is >30%.)
Also know that a fingerstick from an infected needle requires immediate treatment with 3-drug antiretroviral therapy.

Be aware, the optimal time to initiate therapy is unknown among persons with asymptomatic disease and CD4 count above 200. All decisions regarding starting therapy should be made on the basis of prognosis as determined by CD4 and viral load and the willingness of the patient to adhere to therapy.

Which Combination of drugs to use:

"Strongly recommended" by the CDC:
Use one of the following
  • Efavirenz   • Ritonavir plus indinavir
  • Indinavir   • Ritonavir plus lopinavir
  • Nelfinavir   • Ritonavir plus saquinavir
With one of the following
  • ddI plus 3TC
  • D4T plus DDI (don't use in Pregnant women)
  • D4T plus 3TC
  • ZDV plus DDI
  • ZDV plus 3TC

Note: Ok. You are sweating right? How do you remember all of these? You don't! Just know which combinations NOT to use:
  • ZDV/D4T

  • ddC/ddI
  • ddC/3TC
  • ddC/d4T
This is pretty easy to remember--ZDV plus D4T and ddC combined with any NRTI but ZDV is BAD.

If you are really having trouble—stick with this: Throw out any answer that has:
  • ZDV/D4T combined
  • ddC anywhere in the choice
  • Single drug therapy

  and you are probably correct! Otherwise you can combine these drugs into multiple permutations!

When to change HIV therapy:

This is again controversial. However 2 things to know:
  1. Don't change drugs based on 1 viral load; always repeat a high viral load to be sure it is not lab error.
  2. Intolerance to the medication should prompt evaluation for change of therapy.

Possible reasons to change therapy are based on Treatment failure (various definitions and not standardized):
  • Therapy has not suppressed viral RNA to undetectable levels (< 50 copies) within 4-6 months of starting therapy
  • An increase of 3 or more fold from the nadir of plasma HIV RNA
  • Previously undetectable levels now surpassing 5-10,000 copies

The other problem is what drug to change to? Generally just know you should probably change therapy based on resistance testing.

Postexposure prophylaxis (PEP)

First determine the exposure risk: Was the source material blood or bloody fluid? If so, then determine was it a percutaneous exposure (yes—PEP recommended), mucous membrane or skin with compromised integrity (PEP probably recommended). It is easier (and frequently asked on tests) to remember who NOT to give PEP too: Do NOT give for intact skin exposures and urine source exposures. The current thought is to use potent combination therapy. Treatment should start ASAP—within hours of exposure. The standard regimen is ZDV, 3TC, +/- Indinavir/nelfinavir.

Pregnancy

At this time, ZDV is the only drug recommended to prevent "vertical" transmission of HIV. Optimally the mother should receive ZDV as one of her HAART drugs as well as receive intravenous ZDV during labor and delivery. Newborns are treated and, if possible, bottle-fed instead of breast-fed.
Most experts recommend that pregnant HIV+ patients receive highly active anti-retroviral therapy (HAART) just as nonpregnant patients do.

notes

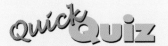

1) Is this a good drug combination for someone with HIV? ZDV/D4T/Indinivir.

2) A patient presents on the examination with *Pneumocystis* pneumonia and HIV. Once she is stable would you start her on anti-retroviral therapy?

3) A health care worker spills HIV-infected urine on their ungloved hand while changing a Foley bag—should they receive prophylaxis against HIV?

4) What is the treatment for PCP in an AIDS patient that presents with a PaO2 of 50?

Suppressing the viral load in the mother likely lowers the risk of transmission to the newborn. New data from developing countries has shown nevirapine, if given during late pregnancy or at the time of delivery, is effective in preventing transmission to the baby.

The bottom line for most pregnant women—treat them with HAART, include ZDV if possible and do NOT use efavirenz (teratogenic) or a D4T/ddI combination (increased risk of lactic acidosis in pregnant women).

HIV ASSOCIATED INFECTIONS AND CONDITIONS:

Introduction

Signs of HIV disease include persistent or recurrent seborrheic dermatitis, *Taenia* infections, psoriasis, molluscum contagiosum, folliculitis, and mucocutaneous infections (hairy leukoplakia, herpes, oral or vaginal candidiasis). Know these. Hairy leukoplakia is caused by EBV. [pg 1-3, #1-9]

Kaposi lesions are a neoplasia of blood vessels and are due to Human Herpesvirus 8. Lesions are heaped up and well localized, often with some surrounding bruising.

Don't forget the Acute Retroviral Syndrome: This is a flu or mononucleosis-like syndrome that occurs 2-4 weeks after initial infection and lasts 1-2 weeks. Patients present with fever, lymphadenopathy, pharyngitis, rash (usually erythematous maculopapular with lesions on face, trunk or extremities including palms and soles), mucocutaneous ulcerations involving the mouth, esophagus or genitals and myalgias/arthralgias. Consider it in a young person who has multiple sexual partners/IV drug user and presents with signs/symptoms of mono or scarlet fever.

Know that you can do a coronary artery bypass (CABG) on an HIV patient if they have a > 10 year prognosis.

PCP and HIV

Pneumocystis carinii pneumonia (PCP [pg 2, #6]) is the most common opportunistic infection in AIDS patients. It is the presenting illness in 50% of AIDS patients. It is probably the most common lung infection overall in these patients but, because prophylaxis is so effective, PCP incidence in AIDS patients is decreasing to less than that of *S. pneumonia* in some places.

Presentation of PCP: insidious onset of fever, shortness of breath, dry cough. ABG: pH > 7.40. A-a gradient is wide. Hypoxia is common. PCO_3 is low (from respiratory alkalosis). LDH is elevated (> 400) and liver enzymes are normal. The Chest x-ray usually shows a diffuse "batwing" infiltrate, although it may also be lobar or unilateral. Occasionally, the Chest x-ray is normal. Again, PCP usually has an insidious onset; if an AIDS patient presents with an acute onset of pulmonary symptoms, first get a sputum for gram stain and C+S and start empirical treatment for community acquired pneumonia. Patients who are most susceptible for PCP have a CD4 count < 200 so all of these patients should be receiving PCP prophylaxis.

The best method of diagnosis is by methenamine silver stain of samples taken by bronchoscopy or BAL, although induced sputum is effective in up to 50% in some hospitals. CMV is usually grown along with PCP from BAL/bronchoscopy samples; only rarely is this significant.

Mild PCP is treated with oral TMP/SMX or atovaquone if unable to tolerate TMP/SMX.

More severe PCP—PO_2< 70 or A-a gradient > 35—is treated with po or IV TMP/SMX or IV pentamidine AND high-dose corticosteroids (which should be started on the first day). Inhaled pentamidine is not recommended for **treatment** of PCP. If there is no response after 1 week or if severe side effects develop, switch. Alternative treatments are dapsone + trimethoprim, clindamycin + primaquine, or atovaquone alone for mild to moderate cases. PCP patients must receive 21 days of effective therapy. Remember to include steroids for any patient with a PO_2 less than 70!

Side effects: Both TMP/SMX and pentamidine can cause neutropenia/leukopenia. TMP/SMX side effects include skin rash, nausea/vomiting, and occasionally fever. Pentamidine causes fever, nausea, vomiting, and diarrhea. Pentamidine also causes azotemia and renal failure. Recurrent courses of pentamidine destroy the islet cells of the pancreas causing hypoglycemia which may not be reversible. (If a patient being treated with pentamidine is found seizing, check fingerstick glucometer!) Hyperglycemia may also occur with pentamidine. Patients on aerosolized pentamidine are at risk for apical pneumothorax. For some AIDS patients, the reactions to either TMP/SMX or to pentamidine are intolerable and the medication must be changed.

Prophylaxis of PCP: give TMP/SMX DS (or SS) one daily or one DS 3 times weekly. If this is not tolerated, give dapsone or atovaquone. Atovaquone has a lower incidence of side effects than TMP/SMX. About 4% of patients discontinue therapy because of rash.

1) TMP/SMX is more effective,
2) TMP/SMX gets extrapulmonary *Pneumocystis carinii*, whereas aerosolized pentamidine does not.
3) TMP/SMX also prophylaxes against toxoplasmosis.

Mycobacterium and HIV

Tuberculosis is also common in AIDS patients, sometimes without infiltrates, and hardly ever with cavitation. Patients usually respond very well to treatment. Do a TB skin test on all persons who are seropositive for HIV. A positive PPD (> 5 mm) without sign of disease is treated with INH for 9 months. Treatment of active TB in a patient with AIDS is the same as in regular patients. See Pulmonology section for treatment.

M. avium Complex (MAC, *M. avium-intracellulare*) is a common infection in patients with AIDS. It is usually disseminated, causing a wasting syndrome with fever, weight-loss, and night sweats. There is no cure. Clarithromycin or azithromycin in combination with ethambutol and sometimes other agents including rifabutin, quinolones, clofazimine, or amikacin can be of benefit in terms of decreasing fever or improving bone marrow function.

Pulmonary: OTHER

Cryptococcus also involves the lung and can be disseminated, but it also commonly goes to the CNS. Cryptococcal meningitis is strongly associated with AIDS, Hodgkin disease, ALL, diabetes, and those who are post-organ transplant. Treat with amphotericin B +/- flucytosine then oral fluconazole. Fluconazole is a good choice for all but critical disease. Flucytosine (5-FC; 5-fluorocytosine) is sometimes not used along with amphotericin B in patients with AIDS because of the problem with bone marrow suppression.

Histoplasma can either affect the lung or disseminate in AIDS patients (only non-AIDS patients have the calcified lung lesions). It can affect many organ systems including the bone marrow. Think of this when an HIV-positive patient presents with interstitial pneumonia, palate ulcers, and splenomegaly and bone marrow suppression. This infection is very common in natives of El Salvador. Treat with itraconazole or amphotericin B. See pg 2-16.

Coccidioides: Again lungs, but it also can disseminate. It is associated with arthralgias, arthritis, hilar adenopathy, erythema multiforme, and erythema nodosum (similar to sarcoidosis). Treatment suppresses, but usually does not cure, this disease, so chronic suppressive treatment is needed (usually weekly fluconazole—1st choice—or amphotericin B).

Know that both *Aspergillus* (especially associated with marijuana use) and *Mucor* can cause a necrotizing, cavitating pneumonia in AIDS patients.

Pseudomonas infections are seen more in granulocytopenic patients (leukemia, chemotherapy, and post-transplant) than in AIDS patients.

GI and HIV

Organisms to consider in AIDS patients with GI infections: *Candida*, especially with esophagitis. Not all *Candida* esophagitis is associated with thrush. If the patient does not respond to treatment for *Candida*, consider CMV esophagitis. Chronic diarrhea in AIDS patients is usually caused by *Cryptosporidium, Salmonella, Shigella, Cyclospora,* and *Isospora belli. Cryptosporidium* shows up as small round red organisms ("round bodies") against a green background on acid-fast staining of the specimen. There is no effective treatment of Cryptosporidiosis. *Cyclospora* and *Isospora belli* are also acid-fast (*I. belli* is large and oval); both are treated with TMP/SMX.

Neuro and HIV

Subacute diffuse encephalitis (caused directly by HIV) is a common neurologic problem seen in AIDS.

Toxoplasma gondii is most common cause of "AIDS-associated-enhancing-focal-space-occupying-lesions" (but the differential diagnosis also includes CNS lymphomas). CT scan shows CNS abscesses due to *Toxo* as ring-enhancing lesions. They are usually multiple but may be single. If these are seen in any AIDS patient, start empiric treatment for CNS toxoplasmosis: 1) long-term pyrimethamine plus a sulfonamide, 2) clindamycin, or 3) trimetrexate.

Again: for suspected cryptococcal meningitis, get a Cryptococcal antigen test (or India ink) of the CSF or the BLOOD! (more sensitive in HIV patients). Especially consider *Cryptococcus* in the meningitis patient who has AIDS, Hodgkin disease, ALL, diabetes, and those who are post-organ transplant. Treat cryptococcal meningitis initially with amphotericin B, then oral fluconazole.

Syphilis, even if previously treated, may reactivate in AIDS patients and cause neurosyphilis!

Any eye problems are probably due to CMV retinitis (see pg 2-22).

Stopping Prophylaxis Guidelines

Primary Prophylaxis (NO history of these infections)
PCP: If CD4 > 200 for 3 or more months in response to HAART can discontinue PCP prophylaxis.
MAC: If CD4 > 100 for 3 or more months in response to HAART can discontinue MAC prophylaxis

notes

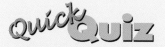

Secondary Prophylaxis (+ History of these infections)

PCP: If CD4 > 200 for 3 or more months in response to HAART can discontinue PCP prophylaxis

MAC: Controversial on whether if and when you can stop MAC prophylaxis with a history of MAC

COMMON ID SYNDROMES

HEART: Bacterial Endocarditis

Introduction

Bacterial Endocarditis—See Cardiology section for prophylaxis indications and medications. See Table 2-4 for treatment and diagnosis. Blood cultures are vital in diagnosing endocarditis of any type and should be drawn before empiric antibiotics are started. Blood cultures are usually positive (95%!) due to the constant level of bacteremia. If they are negative (and patient has not been partially treated with antibiotics), then think of fungi, Q fever (*Coxiella burnetii*), *Legionella*, *Chlamydia psittaci*, and the HACEK organisms (discussed below) as possible causes. Surgery is required for endocarditis with fistula, abscess, pericarditis, or persistent fever, and for cases in which the resulting valve dysfunction causes ventricular failure. In the heart, the electrical conduction pathway passes just beside the aortic valve; a conduction disturbance in a patient with aortic valve endocarditis is another indication for surgery. Vegetations alone usually are not an indication for surgery.

Again: CHF with endocarditis is an indication for cardiac surgery and mortality in endocarditis surgery correlates with the preop severity of ventricular failure. The most common cause of cardiac death due to endocarditis is congestive heart failure.

ABE vs. SBE

There are two methods of classification of endocarditis. The classic method is based on acuity of presentation: acute vs. subacute. The more recent method is based on pertinent etiologic factors: Native valve, Prosthetic valve, Addict (i.e., IV drugs), and Culture-negative. These may have acute or subacute presentations. Addict and culture-negative can also be thought of as subsets of native valve and prosthetic valve endocarditis. In Table 2-4, they are shown only as subsets of native valve because this is the setting in which they generally occur. The distinction is important because the frequency of occurrence of the various organisms is different in each group.

In acute native valve endocarditis, *S. aureus* is the most common cause (40%). Next in frequency is pneumococcus, and then Group A streptococcus. All of the streptococcal infections = 35%. The following occur with about 5% frequency each: enterococci, gram-negative organisms, and *S. epidermidis*.

Overall (acute and subacute), the major organisms are *S. aureus* and viridans group streptococci.

In addicts, the major organism is again *S. aureus* (50%), followed by enterococci (15%). The following 3 have a frequency of 7-8% in this group: strep, gram-negative (usually *Pseudomonas* or *Serratia*), and candida.

In prosthetic valve endocarditis occurring up to 1 year after surgery, by far the most common organism is *S. epidermidis*, (55-60%).

Acute bacterial endocarditis (ABE) is caused by virulent bacteria, often attacking normal valves. It has an acute course in which there is often rapid cardiac valve destruction and resultant ventricular decompensation. There is about 50% mortality with *Staph aureus* endocarditis despite early intervention!

The only common peripheral manifestations of ABE are Janeway spots, which are small nontender macules on the palms and soles. With *Staph*, sometimes peripheral ecchymoses appears. Embolization (again, especially with *S. aureus*) of the heart vegetations leads to metastatic infection (especially to the CNS and kidneys).

Subacute bacterial endocarditis (SBE) usually occurs in patients with underlying cardiac disease. Manifestations include low grade fever, heart murmurs, conjunctival petechiae, splenomegaly (in 2/3), splinter hemorrhages, Roth spots, and Osler nodes.

Roth spots are pale retinal lesions surrounded by hemorrhage. Osler nodes (= OUCHlers nodes) are ~ 0.5 cm tender nodules found on the palms, fingertips, and soles. Roth spots and Osler nodes are late developments of SBE and are seen less frequently today as SBE is diagnosed and treated earlier. Remember that the Janeway lesions (nontender macules) are found in ABE, usually not SBE.

notes

Native Valve

Native valve SBE is more common on the left side of the heart and usually occurs on regurgitant AV valves (although it can also occur with VSDs and PDAs). Mitral valve prolapse is the most common valve lesion associated with native valve SBE! Prosthetic valve endocarditis is seen even more often. *Strep viridans* (from the oropharynx) is the most common cause of SBE, then enterococcal group D Strep (GI, urinary tract), then non-enterococcal group D Strep. In SBE, embolization of the heart vegetations only rarely lead to metastatic infection.

Strep bovis, one of the group D streptococci, is the only type that is easily killed by PCN alone. The other non-enterococcal group D strep require an aminoglycoside plus a beta-lactam antibiotic (two 'cidal antibiotics). Enterococcal group D strep requires ampicillin and gentamicin (not streptomycin). This is why the empiric treatment for endocarditis usually includes naf/ox (for staph) + PCN (required for enterococcus) + gentamicin (for all).

There are some cases of fastidious, gram-negative organisms causing SBE. They are called the "HACEK" organisms (*Haemophilus*, *Actinobacillus*, *Cardiobacterium*, *Eikenella*, and *Kingella*) and usually are sensitive to beta-lactams. These are often the cause of "culture negative" endocarditis, as they may require > 7 days to grow to detectable levels in culture media. Treat with PCN + gentamicin or ceftriaxone or per culture results.

Question: if you see Roth spots or Osler nodes in a patient, what is the treatment? Answer: In SBE, 3-4 sets of blood cultures should be drawn over 24 hours before antibiotics are started. Some elect to wait for the C&S results before initiating SBE treatment.

Also remember endocarditis caused by either *Strep bovis* and *Clostridium septicus* are often associated with colon cancer, so a thorough GI check is indicated in these patients.

Prosthetic Valve

Prosthetic valve endocarditis (PVE) can be acute or subacute in presentation.

Early PVE (< 2 months) is usually due to seeding during the surgery. An acute presentation means emergent surgery is necessary. Even with surgery, it still has a 40% mortality.

Late type of PVE (> 2 months) has a subacute presentation. The infection often invades the annulus and surgery is required. *S. epidermidis* is the culprit in 55-60% of the cases of PVE in the first year after surgery. If the infecting organism is *Strep viridans*, the prosthetic valve infection may be cured with antibiotics alone.

Table 2-4: Bacterial Endocarditis – Diagnosis and Treatment – Native vs Prosthetic Valve

DIAGNOSIS AND TREATMENT OF BACTERIAL ENDOCARDITIS						
Classification	Subsets	Presentation	Initial approach	Empiric treatment while awaiting C&S results	Culture results	Normal tx based on organisms (but tx per C&S!!)
Native valve	Non-addict	Acute	*A	1 PCN/amp + naf/ox	*S. aureus* (40%)	(Naf/ox or cefazolin) +/- gent
					S. pneumoniae	PCN G/amp + gentamicin
		Subacute	*S	1. Same as #1 above OR 2. Wait for C&S results before abx tx	*S. viridans*, *S. bovis* (colon cancer!), other strep, enterococcus.	PCN G/amp +/- gentamicin; check for PCN and gentamicin resistance with enterococcus.
	Addict	Acute	*A	Same as #1 above	*S. aureus* (50%); *Pseudomonas*; Other gram neg bacilli (*Serratia marcescens*, *Enterobacteriacea*)	*S. aureus*: same as for non-addict. *Pseudomonas*: same as for *S. aureus*.
		Subacute	*S	Same as #1 or #2 above	*Enterococcus* (15%) Viridans Strep Fungal	*Enterococcus*: Amp + gent; check for beta-lactam and gent resistance. Fungal: amphotericin B + 5-FC
	Culture neg, Non-addict	Subacute	*S	Same as #1 or #2 above.	HACEK organisms (50%)	Amp + gent or ceftriaxone
					Fungal, Also consider Q fever (*Coxiella burnetii*), *C. psittaci*	Fungal: amphotericin B
Prosthetic valve	Early postsurgery (< 2 mo)	Acute	*A	Vanc + gent + rifampin	*S. epidermidis* (55-60%)	Vanc + gent + rifampin for 14 days then vanc + rifampin for 4 wks.
					S. aureus, Strep, cult neg (each <10%)	*S. aureus*: (Naf/ox or cefazolin) +/- gent
	Late postsurgery (> 2 mo)	Subacute	*S	Vanc + gent + rifampin	*S. epidermidis* (55-60%) Viridans Strep *S. aureus*	Vanc + gent + rifampin for 14 days then vanc + rifampin for 4 wks.

*A: Draw 1st set of BC and start empiric tx. Note: Acute presentation often includes Janeway spots.
*S: Draw 3-4 sets of blood cultures over 24 hours and then initiate empiric treatment (some physicians elect to wait for results with subacute presentation.). Note: Subacute presentation, if caught late, may include Osler nodes and Roth spots. Note: SBE suggests a preexisting valvular abnormality. The above antibiotics give you a general feel for the treatment but there are many other equally valid treatments.
Note: If PCN allergic, give ceftriaxone or vancomycin for PCN-sensitive; vancomycin for PCN-resistant; Vanc + gent for enterococcus; vanc for S. aureus.

notes

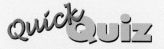

1) What is the treatment for S. bovis native valve endocarditis?

2) What should you look for in a patient with S. bovis endocarditis?

3) When are antibiotics given for patients with suspected meningitis?

4) A cranial nerve palsy should make you think of which 2 types of meningitis: (Hint: One is a spirochete and the other is a Mycobacterium.) Which antibiotics are given for empiric treatment of meningitis?

5) What do gram-negative intracellular diplococci imply in a smear of a discharge from urethritis?

6) What is the most common cause of bacterial meningitis in the United States?

7) What is the treatment for Streptococcus pneumoniae meningitis?

Treatment of Bacterial Endocarditis

Treatment of native valve endocarditis:

1) PCN-sensitive streptococcus (*S. bovis*): 2 weeks of PCN G or ampicillin + gentamicin or 4 weeks of either PCN/ampicillin, cefazolin, or ceftriaxone. Note that, for this, vancomycin is less effective than beta-lactam antibiotics and should be used only for severe PCN allergy. Reliable patients may be discharged from the hospital on a once daily IM dose of ceftriaxone.

2) PCN-insensitive streptococcus (usually *Enterococcus faecalis*): the treatment is 4 weeks of gentamicin plus either PCN G, ampicillin, or vancomycin if PCN-allergic.

3) *S. aureus* endocarditis is treated with oxacillin, vancomycin, or cefazolin; again: if the *S. aureus* is methicillin-resistant, use vancomycin + gentamicin +/- rifampin.

Treatment of prosthetic valve endocarditis:

1) Methicillin-resistant staph (especially *Staph epidermidis*) requires vancomycin, rifampin, and gentamicin—all three—for 14 days followed by vancomycin + rifampin for 4 weeks. The gentamicin prevents the emergence of resistance to rifampin. Remember both gentamicin and vancomycin are nephro- and ototoxic.

2) *S. aureus*: Naf/ox or cefazolin + gentamicin for 5 days followed by the beta-lactam for a total of 6 weeks.

COMMON ID CNS SYNDROMES:

Bacterial Meningitis

Overview

Acute Bacterial Meningitis—If suspected, do the following CSF tests: Gram-stain, C+S, cell count with differential, protein, and glucose.

Previously, CIE (counterimmunoelectrophoresis) or latex fixation were used but they are not cost effective for initial workup—therefore no longer indicated in initial workups. The culture results are the gold standard—unless the patient has been on prior antibiotics. CIE or latex fixation test the following: *H. influenzae*, pneumococcus, meningococcus, Group B *Strep*, *Klebsiella*, and *E. coli*. The sensitivity of these varies from 20% to 90%.

Overall (see Table 2-5), *S. pneumoniae* is the most common cause of meningitis. Next is *Neisseria meningitidis*, and then *Listeria monocytogenes*. > 60 years old is when listerial meningitis becomes more prevalent again.

The main culprit in the meningococcal group is B (B for Bad, B for Bad). There are effective vaccines against A, C, Y, and W-135 but not type B (see pg 2-10 for meningococcemia).

Table 2-5: Etiology of Meningitis in the United States						
MENINGITIS in the U.S.						
0-2 month	%	3 mo to 15 yrs	%	Adult	%	Notes on > 60 yrs
Gram-neg (*E. coli & Klebsiella*)	20-30	*S. Pneumoniae*	30-50	*S. Pneumoniae*	30-50	*S. Pneumoniae* *N. meningitidis*
Strep (Group B) (*S. agalactiae*)	40-50	*N. meningitidis*	10-35	*N. meningitidis*	10-35	See more: *Listeria* *E. coli*, *H. influenzae* *Pseudomonas*
Listeria	2-10	*H. influenzae*	0-7	*Listeria*	2-11	
Staphylococci *S. pneumoniae* *H. influenzae* *N. meningitidis*	2-5 0-5 0-3 0-1	Streptococci Gram Negative Staphylococci *Listeria*	2-4 1-2 1-2 1-2	Gram negative Streptococci Staphylococci *H. influenzae*	1-10 5 5 1-3	
Remember, for the newborn and the adults > 60 yrs, empiric treatment is usually ceftriaxone or other 3rd gen cephalosporin AND AMPICILLIN (cephalosporins have NO effect against Listeria!).						

notes

In neonates (< 1 month old), think gram-negative, group B strep (*S. agalactiae*), and *Listeria*.

In children prior to 1990, *H. influenzae* had been by far the most common cause. The HiB vaccine has had a wonderfully dramatic effect on this disease in the U.S. Its percent of has decreased from about 40% to about 2%!!

Treatment of Bacterial Meningitis

In partially treated gram-positive meningitis, the bacteria stain poorly and they may even look gram-negative! A bloody tap (contaminated) has increased protein and decreased glucose.

Effective treatment requires an antibiotic which both crosses into the CSF and has bactericidal activity.

Antibiotics which cross into the CSF are
- quinolones
- chloramphenicol
- TMP/SMX
- metronidazole

Those which cross into the CSF only with inflamed meninges are:
- PCN
- vancomycin
- 3rd gen cephalosporins
- aztreonam
- imipenem
- clindamycin

Clindamycin has been found to be effective in treating penicillin-resistant pneumococcal meningitis and so probably does cross the blood brain barrier with inflammation. Note that clindamycin is used in the treatment of CNS toxoplasmosis but this is a parenchymal disease and not a meningeal disease, so the drug does not have to cross the blood brain barrier.

Those which do not cross well anytime are
- erythromycin
- tetracycline,
- aminoglycosides
- cefoxitin
- 1st gen cephalosporins

If you see any answers to meningitis questions with these last antibiotics in them, pick something else!

Empiric treatment of meningitis should be started while gram stain and/or culture results are pending. If the LP cannot be done immediately, start antibiotics even before the LP!

- Meningitis in children and adults is empirically treated with ceftriaxone or cefotaxime (3rd gen cephalosporin). But add vancomycin if S. pneumoniae is suspected (e.g., previous antiboitics)!
- For empiric treatment of the elderly and neonates (< 3 months), add ampicillin (for *Listeria*), to the above treatment. So these poor patients are often started on triple antibiotic therapy!

More specifically, in neonates (< 3 mo), use cefotaxime or ceftazidime as the 3rd gen cephalosporin because ceftriaxone may cause hyperbilirubinemia—remember, ceftriaxone causes galbladder sludge in adults).

If you have a suspicion of one of the following, the empiric therapy may change:
- For presumed pneumococcal (especially if gram stain is suspicious) meningitis be sure and add vancomycin to the 3rd gen cephalosporin. Rifampin if vancomycin-allergic.

- Treat presumed meningococcal meningitis with high dose PCN (third-generation cephalosporin if PCN-allergic) and ensure contacts receive prophylaxis.
- The 3rd generation cephalosporins cover gram-negative meningitis.

In AIDS, ALL, or Hodgkin disease, think *Cryptococcus* and do a cryptococcal antigen and/or India ink. Amebic meningitis should be the primary consideration when the meningitis patient has been swimming in brackish (cow ponds) water.

Aseptic Meningitis

Aseptic, chronic meningitis is manifested by headache, meningismus, and CSF lymphocytosis. Many, many causes. On the CSF, do the same tests as for acute meningitis and add fungal serology, VDRL, acid-fast smear and culture, and either the India ink or cryptococcal antigen test. Test results which make aseptic meningitis unlikely are CSF glucose < 40, CSF protein > 150, and CSF WBC > 1200. Viral causes are the most common (hence the most common cause of meningitis) of aseptic meningitis—including enteroviruses and mosquito-borne arboviruses in the summer/early fall, mumps in the spring, and HSV-2 (distinct from herpes encephalitis, which is caused by HSV-1). Suspect *Coccidioides* and *Histoplasma* in endemic areas (arid southwest and Mississippi/Ohio river valleys respectively). A chronic neutrophilic meningitis is unusual—think of *Nocardia*, *Actinomyces*, or fungus as possible causes. Cryptococcus, common in AIDS, Hodgkin disease, and ALL (i.e., cell mediated), is treated with IV amphotericin B + oral flucytosine (5-FC; 5-fluorocytosine) followed by oral fluconazole.

Classic presentation and findings for a viral meningitis: fever, headache, nuchal rigidity, nonfocal exam, normal CT, and an LP showing increased lymphocytes.

TB Meningitis

Tuberculous meningitis is sometimes manifested by cranial nerve palsies, especially the sixth cranial nerve. Other causes of aseptic meningitis include spirochetal (secondary syphilis and Lyme disease).

Lyme Meningitis

Lyme meningitis can cause peripheral and cranial nerve palsies (especially of the seventh cranial nerve) so think of Lyme disease when a patient presents with Bell's palsy and/or foot drop and a suggestive history. Treat meningitis with ceftriaxone 2 gm qd x 21d. Bell's palsy can be treated with oral agents alone. Alternative is high dose PCN G.

Encephalitis

Acute encephalitis—The causes of most of the acute encephalitis cases are unknown! The most commonly identified cause of encephalitis in the U.S. are arboviruses (West Nile, La-Crosse, etc.) HSV is responsible for the highest number of deaths due to encephalitis.

notes

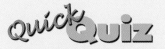

Quick Quiz

1) What are typical LP findings in a patient with viral meningitis?

2) What virus type is the most common cause of acute encephalitis in the US? What virus is the most common cause of death due to encephalitis?

3) Multiple lesions on an MRI of the brain in an HIV infected person should make you think of what organism?

4) What is the antibiotic of choice for diarrhea due to *E. coli* 0157:H7? What about Traveller's diarrhea?

5) How do you diagnose *C. difficile* colitis?

6) How do you treat a recurrent episode of *C. difficile* diarrhea?

Spinal Epidural Abscess

Spinal epidural abscesses may be caused by either hematogenous spread or local extension (from osteomyelitis...). *S. aureus* is the most common cause. Patients present with fever, spinal pain, and nerve compression problems. Do an MRI. CT is not as good as MRI because it is susceptible to bony artifacts. Drainage is required.

Neurosyphilis

Neurosyphilis—also see more about syphilis on pg 2-13. CSF-VDRL test is the test of choice; it is 100% specific, but only 50% sensitive. A positive test confirms neurosyphilis, but a negative test can not be used to rule out neurosyphilis. CSF FTA-ABS is very sensitive—unfortunately, it is so sensitive that a positive result often reflects contamination of CSF with peripheral blood—so it is not used. Often, treatment has to be based on suspicion.

Brain Abscess

Brain Abscess—Diagnosis: CT scan with contrast is the procedure of choice (> 95% sensitivity). If accessible, the abscess is usually aspirated in addition to giving antibiotic treatment. Occasionally need to surgically excise the lesion. Lumbar puncture is absolutely contraindicated if signs of increased intracranial pressure are present—such as focal neurologic signs. Overall the risk of herniation is as high as 20%

Cysticercosis (caused by ingesting the pork tapeworm, *Taenia solium*) is the most common cause of brain lesions in developing countries, and imported cases are often seen in the US. Symptoms, especially seizures, are seen when the cysticerci (larval forms of *T. solium*) die, causing an inflammatory reaction. Toxoplasma is the most likely etiologic agent if the patient is immunodeficient—especially if there are multiple lesions—it is usually due to a reactivation of dormant cysts.

Location of the abscess is often related to the source. Frontal lobe—think paranasal sinus: pneumococcus, *H. influenzae*, and anaerobes. Temporal or cerebellum—think middle ear: pneumococcus, *H. influenza*, *S. aureus*, gram-negative. Both frontal and parietal abscesses can be due to hematogenous spread from such things as lung infections and endocarditis.

Treatment of brain abscesses is always initially empiric:
- High dose ampicillin or ceftriaxone combined with metronidazole to cover aerobes and anaerobes.
- PCN-allergic: give metronidazole along with a third generation cephalosporin.
- If *Enterobacteriaceae* is suspected (i.e., if ear focus), give a third-generation cephalosporin and metronidazole.
- If there was a neurosurgical procedure, penetrating head trauma, or acute endocarditis, think *S. aureus* and add vancomycin (high incidence of MRSA).

Nocardia pulmonary disease can spread and cause focal lesions in the brain—it is also a rare cause of neutrophilic aseptic meningitis (see just above).

COMMON ID GI SYNDROMES:
Infectious Diarrhea

E. coli is the most common cause of bacterial diarrhea (usually without blood or WBCs) affecting both the resident children and travelers in developing countries. There is an enterohemorrhagic *E. coli* (serotype 0157:H7) which causes localized outbreaks of hemorrhagic colitis, TTP, and HUS (hemolytic uremic syndrome)—usually after eating undercooked beef or unpasteurized milk. Do not treat diarrhea caused by *E. coli* 0157:H7 with antibiotics as you increase the risk of HUS.

Vibrios—think seafood and shellfish. *V. cholerae* 01 (causes cholera) is occasionally associated with Gulf coast crabs. The *non*-01 *V. cholera*, *V. parahaemolyticus*, and other *Vibrios* are even more frequent causes of shellfish- associated diarrhea. These are usually self-limited. *Vibrio vulnificus* causes skin infections and sepsis especially in the setting of immunocompromise or chronic liver disease (see pg 2-38).

Fecal WBCs suggest an invasive-type bacterial etiology and are seen in *Shigella*, *Salmonella*, *Campylobacter jejuni*, *Yersinia enterocolitica*, and amebic GI infections—but remember they are also seen in IBD. All these can be found on C&S and *Vibrios* additionally can be found on stool and O&P. So do a fecal WBC and stool C&S and O&P if you need to workup a diarrhea. See Gastroenterology section for more on diarrhea.

Antibiotic-associated colitis is caused by *Clostridium difficile* (antibiotic-associated diarrhea is usually just a side-effect of the medicine). Symptoms can occur up to 3 weeks after the antibiotics are stopped. To diagnose, do a stool assay for the *Clostridium difficile* cytotoxin. A toxin assay is required because 5% of healthy persons have *C. difficile* in their stool and not all of the *C. difficile* organisms produce the cytotoxin. Treatment: stop the antibiotics and give 7-10 days of metronidazole or oral vancomycin. Other treatments are bacitracin, rifampin, or bile binding resins (cholestyramine...) which bind the toxin. Usual treatment is metronidazole because it is just as effective as oral vancomycin yet much less expensive. Relapse rate on either drug is about 30%. This is usually due to the spores becoming active; just repeat the same treatment! Bacitracin, rifampin, and cholestyramine are used as adjuncts in complicated cases.

Cryptosporidia is known to cause prolonged diarrhea in AIDS patients and a self-limited diarrhea in travelers. It is found with acid-fast stains of the stool (small round red organisms on a green background). Animals (including humans) are the reservoirs.

Travelers' diarrhea is usually caused by enterotoxigenic *E. coli*. Prophylaxis with bismuth subsalicylate (Pepto-Bismol®): two tablets qid (yecch!) or daily quinolone.

Treatment: Mild: Loperamide and single dose quinolone.

Severe: Same except quinolone BID x 3 days.

Note: Start cultures for *Shigella* (usually *Shigella sonnei*!) as soon as possible after the bowel movement because *Shigella* dies soon after exposure to air.

Viral Causes—Rotavirus is frequently found in children. It is the most important cause of severe diarrhea in infants and is easily found in their stools. Norwalk type viruses are associated with clams and oysters causing "winter vomiting disease", but it can also be water borne. Norwalk viruses are identified with the ELISA test.

Treatment—If there are fecal WBCs, do a stool C+S and O+P, but fluoroquinolones or TMP/SMX are usually given empirically although antibiotics may prolong *Salmonella* infection. Do not give antimotility agents for any diarrhea when there are fecal WBCs. *Campylobacter* is resistant to TMP/SMX, so give erythromycin or quinolones instead. Prolonged, intermittent diarrhea with malaise and flatus suggests giardiasis or *Cyclospora*.

COMMON ID SYNDROMES: GU Infections & STD

Note

There are many causes of STD. Know the treatment of all STDs! Many STDs have similar manifestations consisting of genital ulcerations with regional adenopathy (gonorrhea does not have these).

With Genital Ulcerations

Workup of genital ulcer (or ulcers) with regional lymphadenopathy consists of serologic tests for syphilis, culture or antigen test for HSV, culture for *H. ducreyi* (on chocolate agar), and, if indicated by history and physical exam, may need to do LGV titers or biopsy the nodes to look for granulomas (Donovan's bodies).

With syphilis, the ulcer is usually single, clean with raised borders, and painless ([pg 18, #54]; see pg 2-13 for more on syphilis). Syphilis also typically has large painless lymph nodes.

HSV presents with tender grouped vesicles. It may or may not have regional adenopathy. Treat with oral acyclovir for the initial episode; it may also be tried for severe recurrent disease.

Haemophilus ducreyi causes chancroid in which there are tender genital papules which become painful purulent ulcers with irregular borders. There is associated very painful lym-

phadenopathy which rapidly becomes fluctuant and ruptures. Treat with one dose of ceftriaxone (250 mg IM) or oral azithromycin 1.0 gm oral single dose, or ciprofloxacin 500 mg bid x 3 days or erythromycin 500mg qid x 7d.

Lymphogranuloma venereum (LGV) is caused by *Chlamydia trachomatis*. It starts with a painless papule which goes on to ulcerate and then disappears in 1-3 weeks. Inguinal adenopathy develops 2-6 weeks later. In LGV, the adenopathy may bulge over either side of the inguinal ligament and fistulae sometime develop. Usual treatment is doxycycline 100 mg BID x 21 days. Erythromycin 500mg QID x 21 days is active as well.

Granuloma inguinale ("Donovanosis") is rare. *Calymmatobacterium granulomatis* is the causative gram-negative organism which produces terrible looking genital ulcers which are painless! Treat with doxycycline 100 mg BID x 21 days or until well healed—may take 1 month. TMP/SMX also used. Erythromycin if pregnant.

PID

PID can be caused by *N. gonorrhoeae*, *Chlamydia*, and normal vaginal flora (usually anaerobes). Oral contraceptives reduce the risk of severely symptomatic PID caused by gonococci, but "silent" PID has the same incidence of sequelae (infertility...) as does that associated with peritoneal signs! Cervical cultures are not reliable for PID. Occasionally PID patients get a perihepatitis (Fitz-Hugh-Curtis syndrome) with mild LFT abnormalities; this has been caused by both gonorrhea and chlamydia.

Outpatient Treatment: Ceftriaxone 250 mg IM, then doxycycline 100 mg bid x 14 days +/- metronidazole 500mg bid x 14 days. Alternative treatment is fluoroquinolones (both Ofloxacin and levofloxacin are now approved).

Inpatient Treatment: Cefotetan 2 grams IV q 12 (or cefoxitin 2 gm IV q 6) and doxycycline 100 mg orally or IV q 12 hours. An alternative is Clindamycin 900mg IV q 8 hours plus gentamicin. Limited data exists with using IV ofloxacin and levofloxacin but they are also acceptable alternatives with the addition of doxycycline. Again: when treating gonorrhea, always cover for chlamydia. Tubo-ovarian abscess require inpatient intravenous antibiotic therapy-look for the inpatient choices above and note that ampicillin/sulbactam + doxycycline is also recommended for tubo-ovarian abscesses.

Patients treated for chlamydial infections should be followed up with a test for cure at 3 weeks.

Cervicitis

Cervicitis is usually caused by *Chlamydia* (especially if the discharge is mucopurulent), but also *N. gonorrhoeae*, herpes, and papillomaviruses. Because *Chlamydia* is intracellular, you must have cervical cells for a valid smear/culture (so scrape or use a brush). Chlamydia cervicitis commonly has a mucopurulent discharge. Gram stain of cervical discharge is only 50% sensitive for the gonococcus, so a negative smear does not exclude gonococci.

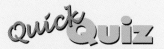

Urethritis

Urethritis—gonococcal or nongonococcal. With GC urethritis, the patient virtually always has a purulent discharge [pg 18, #53], but the diagnosis is made from either positive culture results or the finding of gram-negative intracellular (within PMNs) diplococci on gram stain.

Otherwise, consider it non-GC urethritis, which is usually due to *Chlamydia trachomatis* and, less frequently, *Ureaplasma urealyticum*, *Trichomonas vaginalis*, or HSV. For 35% of cases, the cause is unknown. In the non-GC urethritis, the patients usually have a clear urethral discharge and a gram stain shows WBCs and no bacteria. Gonococcal urethritis has a shorter incubation period (2-6 days vs. 1-4 weeks for *Chlamydia*) and produces a more purulent and more productive discharge.

In all of these patients, check a VDRL and, if negative, repeat it in 2 months (in case the syphilis was incubating when blood for the first test was drawn). HIV testing should be offered to all urethritis patients.

Treatment of urethritis:

1) Non-GC urethritis is treated with azithromycin 1 gm orally in a single dose or doxycycline 100 mg bid x 7 days. Use erythromycin for pregnant women. Azithromycin 1 gm orally x1 appears as effective as doxycycline but it is much more expensive. Levofloxacin and ofloxacin are also effective.

2) GC urethritis. There is about a 20% incidence of gonococcal resistance to penicillin and about the same to tetracycline. Also, because there is often a coinfection with *Chlamydia*, treatment of gonococcal urethritis always should additionally cover *U. urealyticum* and *Chlamydia*. The standard treatment protocol:

  • For uncomplicated gonococcal urethritis or mucopurulent cervicitis, give one dose of cefixime 400mg orally x 1 dose

or ceftriaxone (Rocephin®) 125 mg IM followed by 7 days of doxycycline 100 mg BID or azithromycin 1 gm x single dose. Ciprofloxacin 500 mg, levofloxacin 250 mg, ofloxacin 400 mg and spectinomycin 2 gm IM may be substituted for ceftriaxone in penicillin-allergic patients, but know that spectinomycin does not cure pharyngeal gonococcal disease. Always treat the sexual partners of patients with either type of urethritis, even if they are not symptomatic! And always treat suspected cases immediately—don't wait for C&S results!

Note: There is an increasing trend of quinolone-resistant gonorrhea in Asia. This is slowly moving to the US with incidence of quinolone-resistant gonorrhea at 14% (!) in Hawaii and 0.4% (up from 0.1%) on the West coast (3/2002).

Disseminated Gonococcemia

Disseminated gonococcemia: know! Patients present with a fever, arthralgias, and occasionally oligoarthritis—usually of the knee or ankle. Tenosynovitis is common and frequently asked about. The patient typically has muscle aches and a rash with a few lesions which are papular with hemorrhage into the papules (i.e., very red papules). Notes: Gonococcus-associated arthritis is asymmetric. Gonococcemia is more likely and more severe during menstruation. Pili on the organism are associated with increased virulence.

Gram stain and culture have a very low yield (10%) from the lesions, but if all the orifices are swabbed, there is an 85% yield. Even though the lesions have a low yield, they should still be tested because similar lesions can be caused by other disseminated diseases, such as staph endocarditis (which does have a positive gram stain and C+S).

Patients diagnosed with gonococcemia (including tenosynovitis) should be treated with a 3rd generation cephalosporin (ceftriaxone, ceftizoxime, or cefotaxime) or fluoroquinolones. Pending culture and sensitivity, single-dose azithromycin, ofloxacin/levofloxacin, or doxycycline are included to cover for *Chlamydia*.

Epididymitis

Epididymitis is an inflammation of the epididymis—a convoluted duct on the posterior of the testicle. It is usually caused by infection (know):

  • *Enterobacteriaceae*, especially *E. coli*, in prepubertal boys and men > 35 years old.

  • STD pathogens in sexually active men < 35 years—especially *C. trachomatis*.

Vaginitis

1) Bacterial vaginosis is a clinical syndrome resulting from the replacement of the normal H_2O_2-producing Lactobacillus in the vagina with high concentrations of anaerobic bacteria (Mobiluncus), Gardnerella vaginalis and Mycoplasma hominis. There is a thin, "skim milk", scanty, bad smelling, nonirritating discharge which has two identifying features: clue cells (an epithelial cell with many adherent bacteria) and

notes

a fishy odor when mixed with KOH (+whiff/sniff test). There is no *cervical* discharge. Treatment is usually metronidazole—oral (500 mg BID x 7d) or vaginal gel (.75% BID x 5d). Alternative therapy is clindamycin oral (300 mg BID x 7d) or vaginal cream (2% BID x7d). Treatment guidelines have changed for pregnant women!! Note: Metronidazole 250 mg tid x 7 days or clindamycin 300 mg orally bid x 7 days is now recommended. Creams are NOT recommended in pregnancy. The reason to treat systemically is there is a much higher risk of preterm labor and delivery than complication from a short course of therapy with metronidazole or clindamycin. The male sex partner does not need to be treated.

2) Vulvovaginal candidiasis (VVC) is usually caused by *Candida albicans*. It presents with adherent white plaques with an erythematous base [pg 15, #45]. Treatment:

• Uncomplicated VVC in a non-pregnant patient: clotrimazole or miconazole OTC vaginal creams or clotrimazole 500 mg tablet intravaginally are the least expensive effective treatments. Oral azoles are equally effective—especially oral fluconazole 150mg one time dose!

• The pregnant patient should be treated only with the azole creams for 7 days.

• A subgroup of patients have recurrent VVC which just does not go away and does not have an optimum treatment. Weekly topical clotrimazole or oral fluconazole 150mg one time dose is effective. HIV testing should be done in women with recurrent or persistent VVC.

3) *Trichomonas vaginalis* infection causes a vaginitis in women but men are usually asymptomatic. 1week to 1 month incubation period. Trich vaginitis often presents with a profuse thin frothy yellow-green, bad smelling discharge (which, like bacterial vaginosis, has a + whiff test!), vaginal erythema, and a strawberry cervix. Be able to identify the flagellated organism on wet mount—which is only 50% sensitive. DIF antibody staining is 70-90% sensitive. The vaginal pH is < 4.5 in the normal secretions and in yeast vaginitis. It is > 5.0 in trichomoniasis and bacterial vaginosis.

Treat trich vaginitis with metronidazole 2.0 grams single dose or 500 mg bid x 7d. Even though this is the best treatment, it is only moderately effective. If pregnant, new recommendations say it is ok to give one time dose of 2 gram metronidazole.

Urinary Tract Infection

Acute urethral syndrome (dysuria, frequency, and pyuria) is most commonly caused by *E. coli* and *Chlamydia trachomatis*. *S. saprophyticus* causes cystitis in young women—this is a coagulase negative staphylococcus.

The symptoms of acute urethral syndrome may be due to either urethritis, vaginitis, or cystitis. In women, sexual intercourse can cause *E. coli* to be pushed up the urethra, predisposing them for an acute cystitis. Besides sexual activity, other UTI-predisposing factors in women include spermicide-diaphragm use and an inherited abnormality called Lewis nonsecretor phenotype.

UTIs are rare in men and are not associated with male sexual activity except in homosexuals. In non-homosexual men,

UTIs are usually a result of an abnormality in the urinary tract such as obstruction and ureterovesical reflux from prostatic hypertrophy. Both men and women with DM, neurogenic bladders, or indwelling catheters have an increased frequency of UTIs.

Diagnosis criteria have changed. Urine cultures are no longer required on all young women with symptoms of an acute UTI. If there are no complicating factors, pyuria alone is an indication to treat.

Treatment of UTIs:

• routine UTI: TMP/SMX for three days. (TMP/SMX is more effective than amoxicillin).

• uncomplicated pyelonephritis: the treatment is oral TMP/SMX for 14 days.

• complicated pyelonephritis (including pregnant patients!): IV ampicillin + gentamicin, TMP/SMX, fluoroquinolones, or 3rd generation cephalosporins can be used. Gentamicin alone can be used if the gram stain shows no gram-positive cocci. Follow-up urine analysis after the antibiotic treatment is concluded is recommended. Fluoroquinolones are alternate therapy for complicated or recurrent cystitis or pyelonephritis.

Organisms to know: *Proteus* infections are associated with stones (i.e., do a KUB to check for stones). Group B strep (*S. agalactiae*) infections are seen in pregnancy.

Pregnant: Asymptomatic bacteriuria should be treated in pregnant women (1/3 go on to pyelonephritis!!), neutropenic patients, diabetics, and transplant patients. Also, pregnant patients with pyelonephritis are always admitted and treated as a complicated pyelonephritis (above). Pregnancy-safe antibiotics to use for pyelonephritis are ampicillin, aminoglycosides, cephalosporins, and TMP/SMX but TMP/SMX should not be given in late pregnancy or early nursing mothers because it might cause kernicterus in the child. Tetracycline/doxycycline or quinolones should not be used.

There is an increased frequency of urinary tract infections in patients with DM, SS disease, hyperparathyroidism, or gout. In the last two, the UTI is secondary to stone formation and obstruction. UTIs are the most common nosocomial infections. With normal catheter care, most indwelling urinary catheters stay sterile up to 7 days. They used to be changed after 7 days but it did not make any difference.

Pyelonephritis in older men is often caused by bladder outlet obstruction due to prostatic hypertrophy. Be especially on the look out for *Enterococcus* as well as the usual gram negative organisms!

COMMON ID SYNDROMES: Soft Tissue, Bone, and Joint Infections

Vibrio are found especially in shellfish. *V. vulnificus* causes large hemorrhagic bullae followed by necrosis and lymphadenopathy +/- septicemia. Patients who are immunocompromised or have chronic liver disease are especially susceptible.

Mycobacterium marinum is also called "fishtank bacillus." It causes nonhealing skin ulceration in people who work

notes

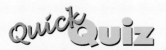

Quick Quiz

1) In a healthy young woman what is the length of therapy for a routine UTI?

2) Asymptomatic bacteruria is always treated with antibiotics in which group of patients? Why?

3) What type of bacteria are commonly found in shellfish? Who are especially susceptible?

4) Acute osteomyelitis is usually caused by what organism? What organism do you suspect in an IVDA? In SS patients?

5) A patient you suspect has osteomyelitis has a negative bone scan. Do you next do an open bone bx?

6) A fishtank cleaner comes in with nonhealing skin ulcerations in a lymphatic distribution. What is the prime suspect? How is it treated?

7) What is the most common means of spreading infections in the ICU?

around fish tanks. Infection may present as a single granuloma but the organism often invades the lymphatics and can cause a series of lesions over a lymph vessel similar to the lesions seen in sporotrichosis. Lesions tend to localize in the distal extremities because the organism does not grow well at body temperature. DDx: Look for acid fast bacilli in the lesion biopsy. It is treated with ethambutol + rifampin or clarithromycin + rifampin.

Erysipelothrix *rhusiopathiae* is another cause of skin infection in fishermen and meat-handlers. Treat with PCN G, ampicillin, or fluoroquinolones.

Impetigo presents as honey-colored crusts over lesions. *Strep pyogenes* is a common cause, often in combination with *S. aureus*. Remember that *S. pyogenes* also causes scarlet fever, a type of toxic shock syndrome (TSS), pharyngitis, and rheumatic heart disease.

Osteomyelitis—acute vs. chronic. Both have infection, but only chronic osteomyelitis has necrotic bone. Acute is usually caused by *S. aureus*. Think *Pseudomonas* in an IV drug abuser, especially if the infection involves the vertebrae or pelvis. Think *Salmonella* in SS patients. Streptococci are virtually never a cause of osteomyelitis! Blood cultures are usually (2/3!) positive in acute osteomyelitis. A negative pyrophosphate bone scan excludes osteomyelitis, but positive scans are also seen with other infections and with fractures. Usually x-ray changes are only seen with chronic osteomyelitis.

With sinus tract osteomyelitis, C+S of the sinus tract drainage is sufficient if *S. aureus* is found but it is not sufficient otherwise—must use bone biopsy/scraping.

With suspected spinal osteomyelitis, do a needle biopsy as the first diagnostic procedure.

Except for small bone disease, the necrotic bone must be removed before a chronic osteomyelitis can be cured with antibiotics.

Prosthetic Joints—1% get infected. Presentation is usually chronic. X-rays usually show bony changes, but a bone scan may be needed. A joint aspiration must be performed to determine the infecting organism. Coagulase negative Staphylococci (e.g., *S. epidermidis*) are the most common organisms recovered.

COMMON ID SYNDROMES: Nosocomial Infections

Order of frequency: UTI > post-op wound infection > pneumonia.

Nosocomial pneumonia is usually bacterial and has the highest mortality rate of all the nosocomial infections (1/3 if bacteremic... 1/2 if gram-negative bacteremic!). It is usually caused by gram-negative organisms; next most frequently, *Staph aureus*. Resistance may develop quickly if only a single broad spectrum antibiotic is used. If there is an outbreak of bacterial pneumonia (or almost any illness) in the ICU, the most likely vector of transmission is the hands of the ICU workers.

Catheter-related infections—there are three types, and all three can cause bacteremia/fungemia: 1) asymptomatic, 2) localized, and 3) septic thrombophlebitis (rarest—see *Candida* on pg 2-15). Secondary endocarditis is more likely to occur in patients with catheters that extend into the heart. IV lines become infected after about three days! Metal needles are less likely than plastic angiocatheters to become infected. IV catheter infections are usually due to *S. epidermidis* and *S. aureus*. Some other causes are *Candida*, *Corynebacterium jeikeium* (especially in bone marrow transplant units) and gram-negative rods.

Treatment: remove catheter and give antibiotic therapy for 2 weeks. Septic thrombophlebitis often requires removal of the affected vein. If there is gram-positive septicemia, start with vancomycin in case it is methicillin-resistant. Exception—if there is a gram-positive bacteremia in a patient with a Hickman or Broviac, you can try to treat with antibiotics for 2-4 weeks without removing the catheter. Again, start with vancomycin until culture results are back.

notes

These questions are to assist you in integrating the information you have just reviewed in this section. These are purposely NOT board-style questions as they are meant to cover a lot of material in minimal space. MedStudy does have board-style Q&As in books and CD-ROM format.

SINGLE BEST ANSWER

1) A. Infections caused by Nocardia and Listeria, fungi, and protozoa.
   B. Infections from encapsulated organisms (*H. flu*, pneumococcus, meningococcus).
   C. Asthma and recurrent pneumonia.
   D. Infections caused by gram negative organisms, *S. aureus*, and fungi.
   E. None of the above.

Which of the following cause an increased tendency for the above infections?

1. Splenectomy.
2. Neutropenia/granulocytopenia.
3. C1 deficiency.
4. C8 deficiency.
5. Multiple myeloma.
6. IgA deficiency.
7. T-cell deficiency

[1(B. This is effectively a humoral deficiency. Babesiosis and malaria are also much worse in splenectomized patients.) 2(D) 3(B) 4(B. Same infections are seen in humoral deficiency. Patients with late complement deficiency are especially susceptible to meningococcal infections.) 5(B; MM causes a humoral deficiency) 6(C; IgA deficiency also is suggested with recurrent giardiasis.) 7(A)]

2) Post-transplant infections
   A. Within first month post-transplant
   B. Within 6 weeks post-transplant
   C. 1-4 months post-transplant
   D. 2-6 months post-transplant
   E. After 4 months post-transplant

1. Cryptococcus neoformans.
2. Nosocomial infections.
3. T-cell deficiency associated infections.
4. Viruses.
5. HSV reactivation.

[This is a set of questions in which there is more than one answer for many of the questions but you must pick the single best answer. 1(E) 2(A) 3(C; especially CMV) 4(D; The viruses are also due to T-cell deficiency but all except CMV tend to occur a little later than the other T-cell deficiency infections.) 5(B; this overlaps with the nosocomial infections but is easy to differentiate.)]

3) Infections caused by gram-positive organisms:
   A. *Staph aureus*
   B. *Staph epidermidis*
   C. *Strep pyogenes*
   D. *Strep pneumoniae*
   E. *Strep agalactiae*
   F. *Enterococcus faecalis*
   G. *Listeria monocytogenes*
   H. *Corynebacterium diphtheriae*
   I. *Corynebacterium jeikeium* (JK)
   J. *Bacillus anthracis*
   K. *Bacillus cereus*
   L. *Clostridium septicum*

1. Painless black eschars.
2. Sepsis after a TURP.
3. Severe resistant infection seen in bone marrow transplant units.
4. Associated with GI malignancy.
5. Most common cause of bacteremia after prosthetic valve surgery.
6. Most common cause of bacteremia in IV drug abusers and dialysis patients.
7. Most common cause of IV catheter-related bacteremia.
8. Pharyngitis with high grade fever, tender cervical lymphadenopathy, and exudative tonsils.
9. M protein.
10. Alpha toxin.
11. TSS with negative blood cultures.
12. Hoarseness, sore throat, and low-grade fever.

[1(J) 2(F) 3(I) 4(L) 5(B) 6(A) 7(B) 8(C) 9(C. The major protein on the *S. Pyogenes* cell surface is the "M protein." The M protein defines which strains are rheumatogenic, cause glomerulonephritis, toxigenic for toxic shock syndrome, etc.) 10(L and all other Clostridia) 11(A) 12(H)]

4) Infections caused by acid-fast bacteria:
   A. *M. avium-intracellulare*
   B. *M. marinum*
   C. *M. tuberculosis*
   D. *Nocardia asteroides*
   E. *Cryptosporidium*
   F. *Isospora belli*

1. Pleural effusion has a high lymphocyte count, no bacteria, and a low glucose.
2. Associated with thin-walled cavitary lung lesions and brain lesions.
3. Causes strings of nonhealing ulcers over lymph channels.
4. Common cause of chronic diarrhea in AIDS patients. Small and round.
5. Lymphadenitis in children.
6. Common cause of chronic diarrhea in AIDS patients. Large and oval.

[1(C) 2(D) 3(B; this is called the "fishtank bacillus.") 4(E) 5(A; as does *M. scrofulaceum*) 6(F)]

5) Match the facts with the following diseases:
   A. Brucellosis
   B. Tularemia
   C. Plague
   D. Bartonellosis
   E. Legionellosis
   F. Typhoid fever
   G. Rocky mountain spotted fever
   H. Leptospirosis

1. Presenting symptoms: pneumonia, confusion, and diarrhea.
2. Carriers of this disease often have seeding in the gallstones.
3. Maculopapular to petechial rash. Fever and arthralgias.
4. Causes abortions in affected cattle; does not cause abortions in humans.
5. Hunter gets constitutional symptoms, localized suppurative lymphadenopathy, and no skin signs.
6. Hunter gets constitutional symptoms, localized lymphadenopathy, and localized ulceration and diffuse rash.
7. Suspect this in a hepatitis with the bilirubin disproportionately high compared to the liver enzymes.
8. Rapid onset of febrile hemolytic anemia.

[1(E) 2(F) 3(G) 4(A) 5(C) 6(B) 7(H) 8(D)]

6) Syphilis
   A. Primary infection
   B. Secondary infection
   C. Tertiary infection.
   D. None of the above

1. Variable mucocutaneous lesions.
2. Diffuse involvement.
3. CNS lues.
4. Painless chancre.
5. Lesions on the palms and soles.
6. General lymphadenopathy.
7. Aortitis.
8. Argyll Robertson pupil

[1(B) 2(B. Secondary infection is characterized by diffuse rash, lymphadenopathy, meningovascular disease, etc.) 3(C) 4(A) 5(B) 6(B; the multiple and various skin lesions and generalized lymphadenopathy occur in secondary syphilis.) 7(C) 8(C; CNS disease and aortitis occur in tertiary syphilis.)]

7) Fungi:
   A. Yeasts
   B. Molds
   C. Dimorphic fungi
1. Spores.
2. *Candida*.
3. *Histoplasma*.
4. Dermatophytes.
5. *Cryptococcus*.
6. *Coccidioides*.
7. Most likely to cause systemic disease in the immunocompetent host.
8. *Blastomyces*.
9. *Sporothrix*.

[1(B) 2(A) 3(C) 4(B) 5(A) 6(C) 7(C) 8(C) 9(C)]

8) Fungi:
   A. Dermatophytosis
   B. Chronic mucocutaneous candidiasis
   C. Sporotrichosis
   D. Histoplasmosis
   E. Blastomycosis
   F. Cryptococcal disease. Coccidioidomycosis
   H. Candidiasis
   I. Mucormycosis

1. Pulmonary infiltrates, constitutional symptoms, crusted skin lesions.
2. Interstitial pneumonia, palate ulcers, and splenomegaly.
3. Cotton wool patches on the retina.
4. Associated with a T-cell abnormality.
5. Suspect as a cause of meningitis in an AIDS patient.
6. Skin nodules along the lymphatic channels.
7. Mississippi and Ohio river valleys.
8. Associated with polyglandular deficiency.
9. Black lesion on the nose of a diabetic.
10. Flu symptoms in Arizona.

. [1(E) 2(D) 3(H) 4(B) 5(F) 6(C; remember that patients with this disease often work around soil—e.g., gardeners.) 7(D) 8(B) 9(I) 10(G)]

9) Treatments for parasites:
   A. Chloroquine
   B. Spiramycin
   C. Mefloquine
   D. Chloroquine followed by primaquine.
   E. Pyrimethamine and trisulfapyrimidine
   F. Exchange transfusion followed by clindamycin
   G. TMP/SMX

1. Ocular toxoplasmosis.
2. Duffy RBC antigen.
3. AIDS patient presents with a dry cough and shortness of breath. Chest x-ray shows diffuse infiltrates.
4. P. ovale.
5. AIDS patient with diarrhea. Acid fast stain positive with large oval organisms.
6. P. malariae.
7. Banana gametophyte on peripheral blood smear.
8. Several *Plasmodium* parasites in one cell.
9. Febrile hemolytic anemia in an asplenic patient who is confused and combative. On peripheral smear are intracellular parasites with the form of a tetrad.

[1(E, or Pyrimethamine and sulfadiazine) 2(D; the Duffy RBC antigen is the site of attachment for *P. vivax*.) 3(G) 4(D; Both *P. vivax* and *P. ovale* form hypnozoites in the liver. Primaquine destroys these forms.) 5(G) 6(A) 7(C) 8(C; *P. falciparum* can be treated with chloroquine only if it is chloroquine-sensitive. If not, it can be treated with PO quinine sulfate and either Fansidar, doxycycline, or clindamycin. If the patient is unable to tolerate PO drugs, IV quinine gluconate and IV clindamycin are used.) 9(F; This is babesiosis. Moderate infections are treated with clindamycin.)]

10) A. Giardia lamblia
    B. *Trichomonas vaginalis*
    C. *Trypanosoma*
    D. *Leishmania*
    E. All of the above
    F. None of the above

1. Megacolon.
2. Kala-azar.
3. Protozoa.
4. Duodenal infection.
5. Achalasia.
6. Sleeping sickness.
7. String test.
8. Flagellates.

[1(C) 2(D; Kala-azar is also known as visceral leishmaniasis. It is caused by *L. donovani*.) 3(E) 4(A) 5(C; Achalasia, mega-esophagus, and megacolon can be results of *T. cruzi* infection.) 6(C; *T. brucei* is transmitted via the tsetse fly.) 7(A) 8(E; The flagellates, which include all of the above organisms, are a type of protozoa.)]

---

11) Helminths: Trematodes (flukes)
    A. *Clonorchis sinensis*
    B. *Schistosoma haematobium*
    C. *Schistosoma mansoni*
    D. *Schistosoma japonicum*
    E. All of the above
    F. None of the above

1. Infects the bladder.
2. Caused by eating raw fish; causes biliary obstruction.
3. Found in Asia.
4. Found in South America.
5. Endemic in Japan and Korea.

[1(B) 2(A) 3(A,D) 4(C; also in Africa and the Middle East) 5(A)]

---

12) Helminths: Nematodes
    A. *Ascaris lumbricoides*
    B. *Enterobius*
    C. *Necator americanus*
    D. *Trichuris*
    E. *Trichinella spiralis*
    F. *Wuchereria bancrofti*
    G. *Strongyloides*

1. Rectal itching.
2. Replicates in the body.
3. Elephantiasis.
4. Frequency of infection in the U. S. is 4%.
5. Roundworm.
6. Pinworm.
7. Infection often lasts for decades.
8. Hookworm. Causes weakness and fatigue.
9. Whipworm.
10. Organism is usually found in pork.

[1(B) 2(G; *Strongyloides* is virtually the only helminth which replicates in the body.) 3(F) 4(E; Per autopsy findings.) 5(A) 6(B) 7(G) 8(C) 9(D) 10(E)]

---

13) Herpes viruses:
    A. Herpes zoster
    B. Herpes simplex
    C. Cytomegalovirus (CMV)
    D. Epstein-Barr virus

1. C-section is recommended if mother is shedding at the time of delivery.
2. Chorioretinitis in an AIDS patient.
3. Most common cause of blindness in industrialized nations.
4. Post-transplant patient presents with hepatitis, colitis, encephalitis, and adrenalitis.
5. Heterophil antibody titers positive.
6. Patient presents with altered mental status and left arm paralysis.
7. Atypical lymphocytes.
8. Inclusion bodies.

[1(B; Remember that this is single best answer. The other viruses do not cause an infection which requires a C-section while a vaginal herpes infection at the time of delivery does.) 2(C) 3(B) 4(C) 5(D) 6(B) 7(D) 8(C) Also remember that herpes virus skin infections are diagnosed by finding multinucleated giant cells on the Tzanck test]

---

14) A. Rhinovirus
    B. Respiratory syncytial virus
    C. Parvovirus
    D. Rubeola
    E. Rubella
    F. Hepatitis C

1. High chance of congenital defect if acquired during the first trimester of pregnancy.
2. Koplik's spots.
3. Diagnosed by an ELISA test on nasal secretions.
4. "Slapped-cheek" appearance.
5. Treat with ribavirin.
6. Measles.
7. German measles.
8. Most common cause of URIs.
9. Giant pronormoblasts in a bone marrow sample of an AIDS patient with aplastic anemia.

[1(E) 2(D) 3(B) 4(C; This is seen with erythema infectiosum—also known as Fifth's disease) 5(F; Ribavirin is active against hepatitis C in combination with interferon alpha) 6(D) 7(E) 8(A) 9(C)]

---

15) A. Acute bacterial endocarditis
    B. Subacute bacterial endocarditis
    C. Both
    D. Neither

1. Nontender macules on the palms and soles.
2. Pale retinal lesions surrounded by hemorrhage.
3. Tender nodules on the palms, fingertips, and sole.
4. CHF is the most common cause of death.
5. More common on the left side of the heart.
6. 95% of blood cultures are positive.
7. *Staph aureus* is the most common infecting organism.
8. Associated CHF is an indication for surgery.
9. Usually occurs in patients with underlying heart disease.
10. Prosthetic valve endocarditis.

[1(A; Janeway lesions) 2(B; Roth spots) 3(B; Osler nodes) 4(C)
5(B) 6(C) 7(A) 8(C) 9(B) 10(C)]

16) Brain abscess:
    A. *Nocardia*
    B. Pneumococcus, *H. influenza*, and anaerobes.
    C. Pneumococcus, *H. influenza*, I, and gram negative
       organisms.
    D. *Taenia solium.*
    E. *Toxoplasma.*

1. Suspect in frontal lobe abscess.
2. Most common cause in immunodeficient patients.
3. Seeds via a pulmonary infection.
4. Child with history of multiple ear infections presents with
   a brain abscess.
5. Most common cause in developing countries.
6. Suspect in temporal lobe abscess.

[1(B. These organisms are common in sinus infections. Especially suspect sinus origin in a frontal lobe abscess.) 2(E; Especially seen in AIDS patients. Multiple ring-enhancing lesions.)
3(A) 4(C. These organisms are common in ear infections) 5(D.
This organism causes cysticercosis) 6(C. Temporal lobe abscesses are often caused by local extension from an ear infection.)]

17) Diarrhea
    A. *Clostridium difficile*
    B. *E. coli*
    C. *Vibrio*
    D. *Cryptosporidia*
    E. *Shigella*
    F. *Entamoeba histolytica*

1. Liver abscess.
2. Hemolytic-uremic syndrome.
3. Seafood and shellfish.
4. Relapse with this diarrhea is treated with the same antibiotic as used in the initial treatment.
5. Cultures of the stool should be done quickly because the
   organism is fragile.
6. Diagnosed with acid-fast stain of the stool.

[1(F) 2(B. This is *E. coli* serotype 0157:H7.) 3(C) 4(A. This is
because it is usually due to the spores becoming active.) 5(E)
6(D)]

18) Causes of genital ulceration with regional lymphadeno-
    pathy:
    A. Syphilis
    B. *Granuloma inguinale*
    C. Herpes Simplex Virus (HSV) infection
    D. *Lymphogranuloma venereum* (LGV)
    E. Chancroid

1. Terrible-looking painless ulcers.
2. Tender genital nodules which become ulcers. Tender,
   draining regional lymph nodes.
3. Tender grouped vesicles. Regional lymphadenopathy does
   not always develop.
4. Single ulcer with raised border. Painless.
5. Single painless papule/ulcer. Regional lymphadenopathy
   develops after the ulcer resolves.
6. *Chlamydia trachomatis.*
7. *Calymmatobacterium granulomatis.*
8. *Haemophilus ducreyi.*

[1(B) 2(E) 3(C) 4(A) 5(D) 6(D) 7(B) 8(E)]

19) A. Blocks DNA replication.
    B. Blocks supercoiling of DNA.
    C. Blocks transcription of DNA to mRNA
    D. Reversibly inhibits ribosomal synthesis
    E. Irreversibly inhibits ribosomal synthesis

1. Quinolones.
2. Tetracycline, erythromycin, clindamycin, and chloramphenicol.
3. Rifampin.
4. Aminoglycosides.
5. Trimethoprim and sulfonamides.

[1(B) 2(D) 3(C) 4(E) 5(A)]

20) General antibacterial properties of the cephalosporins.
    A. 1st generation
    B. 2nd generation
    C. 3rd generation
    D. All of the above

1. Best of the cephalosporins against beta-lactamase. Especially effective against *N. gonorrhoeae* and *H. influenzae.*
2. Active against *Pseudomonas.*
3. Most Staph, most Strep, not *B. fragilis.*
4. Single-antibiotic empiric treatment for meningitis.
5. Contains the best cephalosporin for anaerobic infections,
   including those caused by *B. fragilis.*
6. Group of cephalosporins which is most effective against
   Staph aureus.

[1(C) 2(C; especially Ceftazidime (Fortaz®)) 3(A) 4(C. Ceftriaxone (Rocephin®), cefotaxime (Claforan®). Remember, if the
patient is newborn, elderly, or pregnant, ampicillin must be added
to cover for *Listeria.*) 5(B; cefoxitin) 6(A)]

CASE HISTORIES

21) A patient presents with fever, diarrhea, diffuse erythema, and hypocalcemia; what condition do you suspect?

    A Toxic shock syndrome.
    B. Red man syndrome.
    C. Scarlet fever.

    [A]

22) If a sheep farmer presents with a history of painless papules which vesiculated and formed ulcers, and he now has non-tender black eschars with non-tender induration and swelling, what would you suspect as the cause?

    A. Leptospirosis.
    B. Brucellosis.
    C. Tularemia.
    D. Anthrax
    E. Plague.

    [D]

23) What causative organisms are suspected in a hunter who presents with constitutional symptoms and lymphadenopathy? Which organism is more likely if this patient also has a rash?

    A. Bartonellosis. Plague.
    B. Plague. Tularemia.
    C. Tularemia. Plague.
    D. Plague. Bartonellosis.
    E. Tularemia. Bartonellosis.
    F. Bartonellosis. Tularemia.

    [B. Tularemia is similar to plague except plague does not cause a rash. Bartonellosis is a disease acquired from sandflies in the Andes mountains. It causes a febrile hemolytic anemia ("Oroya fever").]

24) If a feather-plucker presents to you with pneumonia and splenomegaly, what organism would you suspect as being the cause?

    A. Acute candidiasis.
    B. Psittacosis.
    C. Coccidioidomycosis.
    D. Histoplasmosis.
    E. Sporotrichosis.

    [B]

25) What do you suspect in the patient who presents with the same symptoms but with no history of contact with birds? Use the same answers as the previous question.

    [D. Although *Histoplasma* is found in bird and bat droppings, most people have no history of contact with birds.]

26) A patient who is a frequent camper presents with fever, arthralgias, and a rash which started in the distal extremities as maculopapular but now is petechial. What is the proper treatment?

    A. Tetracycline.
    B. Penicillin VK
    C. Third generation cephalosporin.
    D. TMP/SMX
    E. Clindamycin
    F. Immune globulin

    [A. This patient has Rocky Mountain spotted fever; this can also be treated with doxycycline or chloramphenicol.]

27) If a hiker presents with foot drop, what infectious disease would you consider?

    A. Syphilis.
    B. Ehrlichia canis infection.
    C. Lyme arthritis.
    D. Rocky Mountain spotted fever.
    E. Plague.
    F. Brucellosis.

    [C]

28) A patient presents with a painless chancre on his penis. VDRL is positive. What is the proper treatment?

    A. Benzathine PCN G 2.4 MU IM q week x 3 or doxycycline 100 mg po bid x 4 weeks
    B. PCN G 12-24 MU IV qd for 10-14 days.
    C. Procaine PCN 2-4 MU IM qd with probenecid 500 mg qid for 14 days
    D. Benzathine PCN G 2.4 MU IM or doxycycline 100 mg bid for 14 days
    E. Doxycycline 100 mg bid x 1 month.

    [D. This is also the treatment for the early latency period of secondary syphilis (< 1 year since acquiring the disease). The treatment for late latency of secondary syphilis is given in A. The answers given in B, C, and E are means of treating neurosyphilis; doxycycline is used only if a penicillin-allergic patient cannot be desensitized.]

29) A patient presents with a severe cellulitis of the face. Blood cultures are done and the patient is placed on oral cloxacillin. Two days later the infection appears to be worse. Preliminary results of the blood culture show a coagulase negative Staph. What should be done next?

    A. Nothing, it often takes 2-3 days to notice any change with severe cellulitis.
    B. Repeat blood cultures and change the antibiotic to IV lincomycin.
    C. Repeat blood cultures and change to IV vancomycin.
    D. Repeat blood cultures and change to IV cefazolin.
    E. Change the antibiotic to oral ciprofloxacin.
    F. Change the antibiotic to oral TMP/SMX.

30) An AIDS patient presents with signs and symptoms of meningitis. Which of the following organisms is both a likely cause in this patient and is highly unlikely to occur in an immunocompetent patient?

    A. *Bacillus cereus.*
    B. *S. aureus.*
    C. *Listeria monocytogenes.*
    D. *Cryptococcus neoformans.*
    E. *Corynebacterium jeikeium.*
    F. *S. agalactiae.*

[D]

31) If a diabetic patient of yours presents with a black, necrotic spot on the nose and complaining of headache, what disease entity would you suspect?

    A. Ecthyma gangrenosum
    B. Anthrax.
    C. Rhinocerebral mucormycosis.

[C. Rhinocerebral mucormycosis has a very poor prognosis. Ecthyma gangrenosum (round indurated black lesion with central ulceration) is seen with pseudomonal bacteremia. The cutaneous form of anthrax starts as a painless papule that vesiculates and forms a painless ulcer and then a painless black eschar, often with a lot of nonpitting, painless induration and swelling.]

32) A patient presents one month after an eco-visit of the Amazon rain forests. He is complaining of shaking chills and fever. His family tells you he has episodes of hallucination. His urine shows nephrotic-range proteinuria. What is the treatment for this patient?

    A. Sodium stibogluconate.
    B. Pyrimethamine and sulfadiazine.
    C. Clindamycin.
    D. Chloroquine and primaquine.
    E. Chloroquine alone.
    F. Metronidazole

[E. All the types of malaria can cause nephritis from immune complex deposition. *P. malariae* is the one most commonly associated with nephrotic syndrome. It is usually treated with chloroquine only. *P. vivax* and *P. ovale* require the additional primaquine. Sodium stibogluconate is used to treat Leishmaniasis. Metronidazole: *Giardia, Trichomonas*, and amebiasis. Pyrimethamine and sulfadiazine: toxoplasmosis. Clindamycin: babesiosis.]

33) If a patient presents with a large liver abscess which, when aspirated, shows no amoeba or PMNs, how would it be treated?

    A. Sodium stibogluconate.
    B. Pyrimethamine and sulfadiazine.
    C. Quinacrine.
    D. Clindamycin.
    E. Chloroquine and primaquine.
    F. Chloroquine alone.
    G. Metronidazole

[G. This patient has amebiasis. The *Entamoeba histolytica* is usually not seen in the liver abscess aspirate.]

34) A patient being treated with ganciclovir for a severe CMV infection develops neutropenia and thrombocytopenia. What is the probable cause?

    A. Ganciclovir.
    B. The CMV infection itself.
    C. The combination of the infection and ganciclovir.
    D. It is related to neither the infection nor ganciclovir.

[A. The major toxicity of ganciclovir is bone marrow toxicity (30%!!) resulting in neutropenia and thrombocytopenia.]

35) If a woman who has been pregnant two months presents with a measles-looking rash and the hemagglutination inhibition test is negative, what is the next step that should be done?

    A. Start ribavirin therapy.
    B. Check for inclusion bodies in the skin scraping.
    C. Repeat the test again in 3 weeks.
    D. Give the measles vaccine.
    E. Therapeutic abortion.

[C. The hemagglutination inhibition test is used to diagnose Rubella (German measles). If it is negative in a newly exposed pregnant patient, repeat the test again in 3 weeks (i.e., after the incubation period). If it is then positive, therapeutic abortion is indicated. Ribavirin is used in combination with interferon alpha for hepatitic C. Inclusion bodies found in a BAL specimen are pathognomonic for CMV pneumonitis.]

36) A sickle cell patient presents with extreme fatigue and weakness. Diagnosis is aplastic anemia. The bone marrow biopsy also shows giant pronormoblast cells. What is the probable etiology?

    A. Parvovirus infection
    B. Sickle cell burnout after a nonspecific viral infection.
    C. Acute myelogenous leukemia.
    D. Retrovirus infection.
    E. Norwalk virus infection.
    F. Rhinovirus infection.

[A. Parvovirus infection can cause aplastic anemia in patients with hemolytic anemia or with AIDS. Norwalk virus: winter vomiting disease. Retroviruses: HTLV-1 = T-cell leukemia; HTLV-2 = a T-cell variant of Hairy cell leukemia; HIV = AIDS. Rhinoviruses: main cause of URIs.]

37) A patient presents with a thin "skim milk" vaginal discharge, clue cells, and a positive whiff test. What is the diagnosis?

    A. Bacterial vaginosis.
    B. Yeast vaginitis.
    C. *Chlamydia* infection.
    D. Gonorrhea.
    E. *Trichomonas vaginalis* vaginitis.

[A. Bacterial vaginosis is treated with a 7 day course of metronidazole or clindamycin.]

38) A patient presents with a frothy vaginal discharge, no clue cells, a positive whiff test, and a strawberry cervix. What is the diagnosis?

    A. Bacterial vaginosis.
    B. Yeast vaginitis.
    C. *Chlamydia* infection.
    D. Gonorrhea.
    E. *Trichomonas vaginalis* vaginitis.

[E. *Trichomonas vaginalis* vaginitis is treated with one dose of metronidazole. Notice that both this type of vaginitis and bacterial vaginosis have a positive whiff test but only bacterial vaginosis has the clue cells. Note: buzz phrase for trichomoniasis is "strawberry cervix."]

39) A patient presents with a mucoid cervical discharge. Gram stain of the discharge shows only WBCs. What is the treatment?

    A. Procaine penicillin 2.4 million units IM.
    B. Benzathine penicillin 2.4 million units IM.
    C. Doxycycline 100 mg PO BID for 10 days.
    D. Metronidazole 500 mg PO TID for 7 days.
    E. Ceftriaxone 250 mg IM

[C. The most likely cause of this is *Chlamydia*. Gonorrhea has not been ruled out, but of the choices given, C is the best.]

40) If a patient of yours with a Hickman catheter presents with *S. epidermidis* bacteremia, what treatment is indicated?

    A. Remove the catheter and treat with antibiotics for 7 days.
    B. Remove the catheter and treat with antibiotics for 2-4 weeks.
    C. Leave the catheter in and treat with antibiotics for 2-4 weeks.
    D. Leave the catheter in and treat with antibiotics for 1 month.

[C. This is the treatment for patients with Hickman or Broviac catheters if they have a *S. epidermidis* bacteremia. All other catheters should be removed.]

OPEN-ENDED QUESTIONS

41) What are the three different types of growth factors; how do these substances work?

[Growth factor is the newer name for the substances which include interleukins, colony-stimulating factors, and erythropoietin. These substances are the actual molecules which stimulate the cells by combining with the cell surface receptors.]

42) Another class of cytokines, the interferons, have three types: alpha, beta, and gamma. Which one is the most potent and what cell type produces it?

[The most potent interferon in the immune system is gamma, which is produced by T-cells (both helper and suppressor).]

43) In neutropenic patients on bone marrow transplant wards, *Corynebacterium jeikeium* is an important cause of infections. What is the most common cause of infection in neutropenic patients? What are some of the other causes of infection in these patients?

[Infections in neutropenic patients are usually due to gram-negative bacilli, but *Staphylococcus aureus* is also common and infections due to *S. epidermidis* and fungi (*Candida*, *Aspergillus*, and *Mucor*) also may occur.]

44) Beta-lactam antibiotics are not generally used as the sole antibiotic for neutropenic patients with infection. Why?

[Rapid development of resistance to beta-lactams by gram-negative organisms.]

45) How is it that AIDS patients also have a humoral deficiency?

[The decrease in CD4 cells decreases the normal suppressive effect that CD4 cells have on B cells, and there is an overproduction of nonspecific immunoglobulins—which "gum up the works."]

46) A loss of what organ increases the severity of babesiosis?

[The spleen.]

47) In an atopic patient with frequent bouts of otitis media and giardiasis, what humoral deficiency do you suspect?

[IgA deficiency.]

48) What type of immune deficiency do you suspect in someone with frequent bouts of low grade meningococcemia?

[Late complement deficiency.]

49) In what diseases are patients T cell deficient?

[AIDS, Hodgkin lymphoma, and T-cell ALL. Also patients on steroids or alkylating agents or post-transplant.]

50) What previous infections might reactivate in a person with impaired cellular immunity?

[*Nocardia*, TB, *Cryptococcus*, Blastomycosis, Histoplasmosis, Coccidioidomycosis, and *Strongyloides*.]

51) Name four factors which account for or increase the pathogenicity of the staphylococcus bacteria.

[Enterotoxin, exotoxin, coagulase, and leukocidin.]

52) What type of streptococcal pneumoniae is the most virulent and with what protein is this virulence associated?

[Type 3; M protein.]

53) In what patient groups are you most likely to find an infection caused by *Strep agalactiae*?

[The neonates and the elderly (especially if alcoholic or diabetic).]

54) In what patient groups do infections caused by *Listeria monocytogenes* occur?

[The elderly, neonates, and pregnant women.]

55) What type of infection is most likely after a TURP? How do you treat it?

[Enterococcus. Treat with gentamicin and vancomycin, penicillin, or ampicillin.]

56) In what way is the treatment for *Listeria monocytogenes* infection similar to that for enterococcal infections?

[Both *Listeria* and enterococci are resistant to all cephalosporins. Both are treated with an aminoglycoside and penicillin or ampicillin.]

57) If a patient presents with hoarseness, sore throat, and a low grade fever, what would you suspect as the cause? What if he also had a gray-white pharyngeal membrane? What is the treatment of choice for this organism?

[Viral syndrome. Diphtheria. Erythromycin.]

58) In what situation is *Corynebacterium jeikeium* especially a problem?

[On bone marrow transplant units.]

59) If a patient comes in with sepsis caused by *Clostridium septicum*, what other workup is required?

[GI malignancy workup.]

60) What is the main toxin in all *Clostridia*?

[Alpha toxin.]

61) Name two immune deficiencies in which infection by *Neisseria meningitidis* is more common.

[Humoral deficiencies and late complement deficiencies.]

62) Where does *Salmonella typhi* tend to seed in chronic carriers?

[In the gallbladder.]

63) In what patient group do you expect to see *Moraxella catarrhalis* respiratory infections?

[In patients with COPD and those with immunodeficiencies.]

64) What are buboes?

[Very large lymph nodes (as in bubonic plague).]

65) What type of *Chlamydia* is associated with neonatal eye infections and neonatal pneumonia?

[*C. trachomatis*.]

66) In which type of septic shock does the patient have warm extremities?

[Gram negative.]

67) How long after primary syphilis does secondary syphilis occur? What percentage of untreated secondary syphilis goes on to tertiary syphilis?

[About 2 months. About 33%]

68) Of the two general types of serologic tests for syphilis, the non-treponemal and the specific treponemal, which type is positive in a neonate whose mother was positive?

[Both the specific treponemal and non-treponemal tests are positive.]

69) What organism is especially associated with septic peripheral thrombophlebitis and septic thrombosis of the great central veins?

[*Candida albicans*.]

70) Which antifungal agent is never used for ringworm?

[Amphotericin.]

71) Of the two main types of parasites (protozoa and helminths), which causes eosinophilia? Which are single celled? Which tend to replicate within the body?

[Helminths. Protozoa. Protozoa.]

72) How is the diagnosis of acute toxoplasmosis made?

[Elevated specific IgM antibody.]

73) Which RBC antigen is the site of attachment for *P. vivax*?

[The Duffy RBC antigen.]

74) What does the protozoan, *Babesia microti*, have in common with *Borrelia burgdorferi*? What does it have in common with malaria?

[Both *Babesia microti* and *Borrelia burgdorferi* are transmitted by the *Ixodes* tick. Both *Babesia microti* and the *Plasmodia* are intra-RBC parasites.]

75) What is the only helminth which replicates in the body?

[*Strongyloides* is the only common helminth which replicates in the body.]

76) What is the drug of choice for any type of *Schistosoma* infection?

[Praziquantel.]

77) Which lab result is pathognomonic for herpes zoster infection?

[Multinucleated giant cells in a skin scraping.]

78) Does prednisone given in the treatment for herpes zoster help decrease the incidence of post-herpetic neuralgia?

[It has not been proven to do so.]

79) What type of cells are the atypical lymphs found in a patient with infectious mononucleosis?

[T cells.]

80) How is Epstein-Barr (EB) virus associated with the hairy leukoplakia seen in early HIV disease?

[EB virus +/- papilloma virus causes hairy leukoplakia.]

81) Which virus is ribavirin effective against?

[Ribavirin is treatment of choice for hepatitis C in combination with interferon alpha. It has some activity against Influenza A & B but amantadine, rimantadine, flu vaccine, oseltamivir (Tamiflu®—oral) and zanamivir (Relenza®—powder for inhalation) are preferred treatments or prophylactic agents.]

82) What type of virus are oral amantadine and rimantadine effective against?

[Influenza A.]

83) In a nursing home threatened by influenza A, what should be done?

[The patients, staff, and physicians should all take amantadine/rimantadine and be immunized.]

84) What variants of papillomavirus are associated with cervical cancer?

[16, 18 and 31.]

85) What virus causes progressive multifocal leukoencephalopathy? In what patient group is this usually seen?

[Papovavirus is reactivated in AIDS patients and causes progressive multifocal leukoencephalopathy in this group.]

86) How do you differentiate mumps from bacterial parotitis?

[Gram stain the parotid secretions. Bacterial parotitis has many WBCs in the secretions whereas mumps has none.]

87) What are the CD4 positive cells in which HIV replicates?

[Helper T cells, monocytes, and macrophages.]

88) What causes the polyclonal increase in serum immunoglobulins in AIDS patients?

[The CD4+ helper T cells decrease and no longer tonically suppress the B lymphocytes.]

89) When is antibody to HIV detectable after the initial inoculation? How is this antibody detected?

[Within 2-3 months after the initial inoculation the anti-HIV antibody is detectable by the ELISA test.]

90) What is the significance of the P24 HIV antigen?

[This is an HIV core protein which is an early detectable sign of HIV infection.]

91) What is the most common lung disease in AIDS patients?

[Pneumocystis Pneumonia (PCP).]

92) At what CD4 count is prophylaxis for PCP started?

[< 200.]

93) Which of the drugs used to treat PCP causes neutropenia? Which causes skin rash? Which causes hypoglycemia?

[Neutropenia: TMP/SMX (Bactrim) and pentamidine. Skin rash: TMP/SMX. Hyperglycemia or hypoglycemia: pentamidine.]

94) Why is Fansidar not used much in prophylaxis for PCP?

[Because it (rarely) causes Stevens-Johnson syndrome.]

95) Histoplasmosis or coccidioidomycosis: Which one causes arthralgias? Which one causes splenomegaly?

[Arthralgias: coccidioidomycosis. Splenomegaly: histoplasmosis.]

96) What is the most common neurologic problem in AIDS patients?

[Subacute diffuse encephalitis.]

97) If a patient with AIDS, Hodgkin disease, or diabetes develops meningitis, what test must be done on the CSF in addition to the usual CSF survey?

[Cryptococcal antigen (or India ink).]

98) If the blood cultures are negative in bacterial endocarditis, what organisms are the most likely cause?

[One of the HACEK organisms would be likely: *Haemophilus, Actinobacillus, Cardiobacterium, Eikenella*, and *Kingella*.]

99) When is surgery required in bacterial endocarditis?

[When there is fistula, abscess, pericarditis, or persistent fever, and in cases when the resulting valve dysfunction causes heart failure. Also, when there is a conduction disturbance in a patient with aortic valve endocarditis.]

100) What is the most common cause of death due to endocarditis?

[Ventricular failure.]

101) Name the organisms which most commonly cause acute native valve bacterial endocarditis.

[*Staph aureus* (40%), pneumococci, Group A strep, enterococci, and then gram-negative organisms and S. epidermidis.]

102) What is the only common peripheral manifestation of ABE?

[Janeway spots (nontender macules on the palms and soles).]

103) What are the peripheral manifestations of subacute bacterial endocarditis (SBE)?

[Roth spots (pale retinal lesions surrounded by hemorrhage), petechiae, splinter hemorrhages, and Osler nodes (small tender nodules on the palms, fingertips, and soles).]

104) If a patient presents 45 days after a prosthetic valve insertion and has signs and symptoms of endocarditis, what would be the most likely next step: surgery or intensive medical therapy?

[Early prosthetic valve endocarditis (< 60 days) is usually due to seeding during surgery. It has an acute presentation and requires emergent surgery.]

105) What prosthetic valve endocarditis can sometimes be cured by antibiotics alone?

[*Strep viridans* endocarditis. This usually presents subacutely and > 60 days after surgery.]

106) What organisms do you suspect in a chronic meningitis with a neutrophilic CSF?

[*Nocardia, Actinomyces*, or fungus.]

107) What is the most common cause of acute encephalitis?

[Unknown! Although it is thought to be viral.]

108) What is the procedure of choice for diagnosing brain abscesses? What is the most common cause of brain abscess in developing countries? What is the empiric therapy for brain abscesses?

[CT scan. Cysticercosis (from ingesting the pork tapeworm, *Taenia solium*) is the most common cause in developing countries. See ID section for empiric therapy.]

109) What is the test of choice for diagnosing neurosyphilis? Why is a CSF FTA-ABS not used to diagnose neurosyphilis?

[CSF-VDRL (100% specific, 50% sensitive). The CSF FTA-ABS is so sensitive that a positive result is due to contamination of the sample by peripheral blood.]

110) 5% of healthy persons have *C. difficile* in their stool. How can you tell if the diarrhea is caused by *C. difficile*?

[A *C. difficile* cytotoxin assay is done.]

111) What viruses cause severe diarrhea in infants?

[Rotavirus is the most common cause of severe diarrhea in infants.]

112) What viruses are associated with diarrhea after eating clams or oysters?

[Norwalk virus. This is called "winter vomiting disease." The Norwalk viruses are identified by the ELISA test.]

113) Why is a brush often used in obtaining a cervical *Chlamydia* culture?

[Because *Chlamydia* are intracellular parasites and cells from the cervix are required for diagnosis.]

114) How is gonococcal urethritis diagnosed?

[Positive culture or an exudate gram-stain showing gram-negative intra-WBC diplococci.]

115) What are the causative organisms in non-GC urethritis?

[*Chlamydia trachomatis, Ureaplasma urealyticum, Trichomonas vaginalis*, and HSV.]

116) What is the treatment for non-GC urethritis?

[Azithromycin or doxycycline. Erythromycin if pregnant.]

117) What does the skin rash of disseminated gonococcemia look like?

[It usually consists of a few lesions which are papular with hemorrhage into the papules (very red papules).]

118) What is the best way of making the diagnosis of disseminated gonococcemia?

[Gram stain and C&S of the lesions and all body orifices results in an 85% yield.]

119) How is menstruation associated with severity of symptoms in a GC infection with gonococcemia?

[Severity of symptoms is increased.]

120) What is the pH of the vaginal fluid be in the following situations: normal, yeast vaginitis, trichomoniasis, bacterial vaginosis.

[Normal and yeast vaginitis: < 4.5. Trichomoniasis and bacterial vaginosis: >5.0.]

121) What are the UTI-predisposing factors in women?

[Sexual activity, spermicide-diaphragm use, and Lewis nonsecretor phenotype.]

122) What is the indication to treat a woman with symptoms of acute cystitis and no complicating factors? How does sexual activity influence treatment for UTIs?

[Pyuria alone is an indication to treat in this patient group. If the woman has had many sexual partners, she is given doxycycline to cover for *Chlamydia trachomatis*.]

123) Should asymptomatic bacteriuria be treated in pregnant women? What if it occurs in neutropenic patients? Transplant patients? If there is an indwelling Foley catheter? In a nursing home patient?

[Asymptomatic bacteriuria (> 10^5) should be treated in pregnant patients (1/3 go on to pyelonephritis!), neutropenic patients, diabetics, and transplant patients. It is not treated in elderly patients or patients with Foley catheters.]

124) Why should TMP/SMX (Bactrim®) not be given in late pregnancy?

[TMP/SMX is not given in late pregnancy or early nursing mothers because it can cause kernicterus in the child.]

125) Why do the lesions caused by *Mycobacterium marinum* often localize in the distal extremities?

[Because the organism does not grow well at body temperature.]

126) If an IV drug abuser presents with osteomyelitis of the spine, what is the probable causative organism?

[Think *Pseudomonas* in this patient group, especially if the infection involves the spine or pelvis.]

127) Does a negative pyrophosphate scan exclude osteomyelitis?

[Yes, a negative pyrophosphate scan excludes osteomyelitis. A positive scan can be caused by other infections and with bone fractures.]

128) What is the order of frequency of nosocomial infections?

[UTI > post-op wound infections > pneumonia.]

129) How often should IV lines be changed?

[Every 3 days.]

130) What is the most common vector of nosocomial disease between patients in the ICU?

[Hands of the ICU workers.]

131) What are the common and uncommon causes of IV catheter-related infections?

[Common: *S. aureus* and *S. epidermidis*. Less common: *Candida*, *Corynebacterium jeikeium* and *Bacillus cereus*.]

132) Why is nafcillin used in lieu of methicillin?

[Methicillin is associated with interstitial nephritis.]

133) Why, even though penicillin is the drug of choice for meningococcal infections, is rifampin used for eradication of the carrier state?

[Because it concentrates in the upper respiratory mucosa.]

134) Which is the second generation cephalosporin which is useful in treating meningitis?

None. Only 3rd and 4th generations are now approved for treatment of meningitis.

135) Which of the cephalosporins are active against *Pseudomonas*?

[The third generation cephalosporins, especially ceftazidime (Fortaz®) and cefoperazone (Cefobid®) and the 4th generation cefepime (Maxipime®]

136) Which of the third generation cephalosporins cross an inflamed blood brain barrier?

[Ceftriaxone, cefotaxime, and ceftazidime. Note only ceftriaxone and cefotaxime can be used alone for empiric treatment of meningitis pending results of CSF analysis (if patients are neonates, elderly, or pregnant, ampicillin is added to also cover for *Listeria*). Remember though—if you suspect *S. pneumoniae* add Vancomycin until your sensitivities come back! Ceftazidime does not have enough gram positive coverage anymore to be reliable for any strain of *S. pneumoniae*]

137) Why is ciprofloxacin not recommended for the routine treatment of community acquired pneumonia?

[Because there is concern of *S. pneumoniae* resistance]

138) What are three of the broadest spectrum antibiotics and what are their spectrum?

[Imipenem, meropenem, and cefepime. They are effective against most bacteria. The organisms resistant to them can include *Enterococcus faecium*, *Pseudomonas cepacia*, *Corynebacterium jeikeium*, *Xanthomonas maltophilia*, and methicillin-resistant *Staphylococci*.]

139) Explain the mechanisms of the beta-lactamase inhibitors, sulbactam and clavulanic acid.

[These inhibitors bind irreversibly to the beta-lactamase made by the bacteria.]

140) What is "red man syndrome"?

[Red man syndrome is a NON-ALLERGIC reaction to vancomycin which causes tachycardia, flushing, pruritus, and sometimes angioedema. It results from the release of histamine from mast cells usually because of a too rapid infusion of vancomycin.]

141) Which antibiotics have a persistent anti-gram negative effect after removal of the drug?

[Aminoglycosides.]

142) Which cephalosporin is effective against Listeria?

[None. Penicillin or ampicillin is the drug of choice.

143) Why is doxycycline a drug of choice for community acquired pneumonias?

[Because doxycycline is effective against *Mycoplasma pneumoniae*, *S. pneumoniae*, and *Chlamydia pneumoniae*.]

144) Why is rifampin never given alone to treat an acute infection?

[Because organisms rapidly develop resistance to rifampin.]

145) What is the main toxicity of ganciclovir?

[Bone marrow toxicity.]

146) What are the main side effects of ZDV (zidovudine)?

[Bone marrow suppression, myositis, and hepatitis. With the start of treatment, many patients have nausea, vomiting, and headache.]

147) Why may it be required to discontinue ZDV (zidovudine) when an AIDS patient is being treated for CMV retinitis with ganciclovir?

[Because these drugs have an additive bone marrow suppressive effect.]

148) With amphotericin B, what is the limitation on qod therapy versus qd therapy?

[Every-other-day amphotericin B therapy is just as effective as daily therapy but the qod therapy causes more fever.]

149) What are the side effects of flucytosine?

[It can cause serious GI, hepatic, renal, and bone marrow toxicities.]

150) Ketoconazole is an antifungal drug which has been used to treat Cushing syndrome. What is its mechanism of action in treating Cushing syndrome?

[Ketoconazole blocks the 11-hydroxylase enzyme.]